The Ultimate Massage Chair Buyer's Guide

How to Select the Perfect Massage Chair

For Your Home or Business

Dr. Alan D. Weidner

ISBN: 1499366345
ISBN 13: 9781499366341

Table of Contents

Introduction

The first massage chair was created by a Japanese fellow in the late 1950s. Apparently he was a sewing machine parts manufacturer who had a daughter who suffered from headaches. He made a chair out of sewing machine parts in an effort to create something that would alleviate his daughter's suffering. It ended up helping her and birthing a whole new product and industry.

Massage chair companies started springing up around 1960, with Inada being one of the first. Manufacturing was exclusive to Japan initially, but now chairs are being made primarily in China because of cost advantages.

Massage chairs have become a staple in Japan, if not all of Asia. I have heard figures that 25% or more of homes in Japan have a massage chair. The figure in the United States is quite a bit less than that…perhaps 1% at best. But the massage chair is beginning to take off in North America.

As people become more health conscious and desire to take their health into their own hands, massage chairs will become a more and more popular choice for home health care.

With the increased interest in massage chairs come more massage chair companies, online and offline retailers, chair manufacturers, and, ultimately, increased competition for your hard-earned money.

With all this comes increased confusion over which chair is your best option, let alone if a chair is even something you should consider. You can find literally hundreds of models in the marketplace, but finding the right chair for you is what *The Ultimate Massage Chair Buyer's Guide* is all about.

Some questions that have gone through your mind might include:

1. How can I tell if a chair is a good one or not?
2. Is a higher-priced chair necessarily a better chair?
3. What happens if something goes wrong with my chair?
4. What are the warning signs of a bad deal?
5. Is a massage chair right for me and my situation?
6. What are the contraindications of using a massage chair?
7. What's better, Chinese-made or Japanese-made?
8. Am I too short or tall for a massage chair?

...And the list goes on and on. I have written this buyer's guide to answer all of these questions and many others that you most likely are entertaining or will entertain en route to making the best decision about a massage chair.

Chapter 1 discusses the physiological health benefits of massage, whether that massage is administered by a licensed massage therapist or a robotic massage chair. I think you will be surprised at what a massage chair just might be able to do for your health! I also go into a quick discussion of the advantages of using a massage chair over a licensed massage therapist.

You may wonder if you are a candidate for a massage chair based on your symptoms or complaints. Chapter 2 talks about who could benefit from a massage chair.

Chapter 3 is an eight-point report discussing the most important things you will need to know before deciding on a massage chair. These are things that can make or break your massage chair ownership experience.

What things do you need to consider if you are thinking about getting a massage chair for your business rather than for your home? Chapter 4 goes into detail about some issues you may never even think of that you *must* know before making the buying decision.

Chapter 5 is a discussion of the pros and cons of getting a used or refurbished massage chair instead of a new one. There are some things you really need to know before you take the plunge.

Can your kids sit in the new massage chair? That's a great question that I get asked a lot. Chapter 6 addresses the topic of children and massage chairs.

How about using a massage chair when you are pregnant? This is another popular inquiry from massage chair shoppers, and Chapter 7 deals with it in detail.

A massage chair is not a cheap investment. Chapter 8 shows you how you just might be paying for one already without even realizing it.

Once you own a chair, there are a few housekeeping issues to consider to make your ownership experience a good one. Chapter 9 covers those issues.

Chapter 10 is a little self-serving. Of course, I want you to buy your new chair from Massage Chair Relief. But I don't expect you to buy from us just because I wrote this book. There are plenty of good reasons to buy from us, and I list them all in detail in this chapter.

Don't forget to check out the appendix of the book. There are five very valuable sections that also will assist you greatly in the decision-making process: a) helpful massage chair articles that go into topics not covered in the main body of the book, b) a massage chair glossary to help you understand the industry lingo, c) reviews and testimonials, d) contraindications to massage that you might need to consider before making a decision, and e) massage chair resources available to you.

Massage chairs are not cheap to buy, and if you choose to return your chair, shipping can be astronomical. You want to make the most educated decision you can when shopping for a chair so that you feel good about your investment throughout the whole buying and ownership process. I have written this book to that end. I want this book to make your journey of finding the perfect home health care therapy a joyous and rewarding one. Now...let's begin!

Chapter 1

Health Benefits of Massage Therapy

Massage therapy has been around for millennia and will, no doubt, be around for many more. What is it about massage therapy that is so appealing? Is it just because it feels so dang good to have it done to you, or is there more to it? Are there actual therapeutic benefits that truly enhance your health? And what about robotic massage chairs specifically? Can they offer something that enhances your overall health and well-being?

Well, the answer to these questions is a resounding *yes!* I am going to present a list of therapeutic benefits that come from massage therapy, along with some details about how they will affect you. Although this is an e-book about massage chairs per se, the benefits of massage are, of course, available through robotic massage chairs as well as manual, hands-on massage from a licensed massage therapist.

The list of health benefits from massage therapy, including from a robotic massage chair, is going to surprise you. It is a lot longer and more comprehensive than you would have ever imagined. As far as massage chairs go and their application of massage therapy, if you think a massage chair is just an elaborate and lovely electronic gadget that only the rich indulge in, you've got another think coming. It is so much more than just *ooohhh* and *aaahhh!* There are many reasons to use a massage chair:

- One of the many great benefits of massage is the wonderful therapy it provides to your tired, tight, and aching muscles. No matter what type of job you perform each day, any repeated action creates sore, stiff muscles. Individuals who work in an office sit and look at a computer all day. Even the action of sitting is still extremely stressful on many muscles, ligaments, nerves, and bones throughout the body, especially in the neck and back regions. Those who perform manual labor suffer stiffness in many of these same areas. Even those who drive a school bus or a delivery truck experience musculoskeletal soreness.

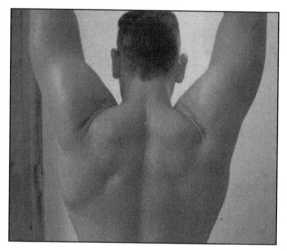

Massage can loosen all of these stiff, aching muscles. The kneading and tapping of massage creates heat by increasing blood flow to the tissues being massaged. This allows the muscles to relax completely for deeper penetration. Many people say they feel like a limp rag doll after just one massage session.

- It's not at all uncommon today for people to have trouble falling asleep after spending all day at work. It is difficult to doze off with the weight of the world upon your shoulders, especially if it feels as if you've have been carrying that weight all your life. A massage therapy session will loosen muscles and relax your body, making it much easier to fall asleep. Being relaxed allows you to find a comfortable position to rest your weary body and *stay* asleep.

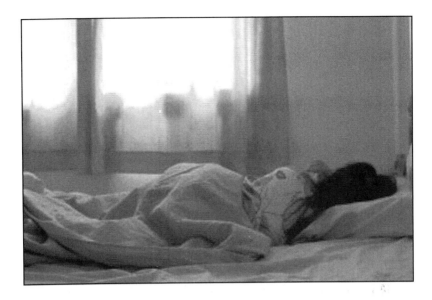

- Overuse of muscles can lead to horrible chronic back and neck pain. And these pains are the same for everyone... regardless of your profession, overuse syndromes can and do occur. One day or one week of being in the same position performing the same activities for eight hours or more each day will make a person stiff and sore. Continuing to do so for years with no relief can lead to muscle hypertonicity and, ultimately, muscle strain injuries. Regular massage sessions will reduce the soreness and prevent injuries. Muscle strains that go on untreated may even result in a need for surgery or toxic medicines in order to find some pain relief. Massage therapy is a safe, holistic method to treat muscle strain.

- One of the surprising benefits of a massage chair is that it promotes proper posture! Improper posture is one of the leading causes of not only neck and back pain, but also neck and back injuries. Poor posture does not just damage muscles; it severely damages ligaments and bones as well. When we were children, our parents usually reminded us to stand and sit correctly. As we become adults, we get caught up in the hustle and bustle of life, not to mention the strain of a job that promotes poor posture, and sometimes we forget these instructions. Massage chair therapy reminds our bodies that it feels wonderful to sit and stand correctly. After a session in a massage chair, you will arise from the chair feeling taller and straighter. Some chairs even employ airbags that put your body in a proper posture position. Many times when you are suffering from sore muscles, it may be too painful to stand or sit properly. Beginning this type of massage regimen will encourage your muscles to relax and make it possible for you to stand proud and tall once again.

- Encouraging yourself to sit and stand with proper posture can also reduce further nerve damage and the pain of existing nerve damage. Through incorrect positioning and unnecessary stress on muscles and bones, pressure on our nerves increases. While muscle and bone stress is extremely painful, many individuals believe that nerve pain is worse. Massage therapy may reduce stress on these nerves and even decrease the pain associated with a neuropathy.

- Massage therapy can slow down the process of degenerative arthritis and alleviate associated pain. Part of this is due to the fact that it promotes proper posture. Through poor posture, we put too much unnecessary stress on our bones. This adversely affects these bones and the surrounding soft tissue, resulting in degenerative types of arthritis. Granted, if you are over 40 years of age, you have already begun to feel this type of pain and stiffness. Arthritis is no longer an older adult disorder. People of any age can suffer from different types of arthritis because of continued poor posture, sports-related injuries, or bone and muscle disorders.

Another way a massage chair can slow arthritic degeneration is by offering passive motion to spinal joints that ordinarily would not get any attention through exercise or other treatments. These neglected joints are the ones that typically develop degenerative changes.

• Massage therapy has some of the same benefits as practicing yoga. Most individuals begin the practice of yoga to become more flexible and teach the body to breathe properly. Sessions in a massage chair will greatly increase your flexibility. This can be demonstrated by performing a simple test. Before sitting in the massage chair, try touching your toes or bending forward as far as you can. Once the session is complete, try this again. You will notice a dramatic increase in your flexibility…and that's after only a single session! This is because of how much massage relaxes the muscles and allows them to rest.

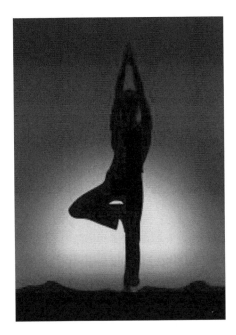

• Massage therapy promotes better breathing. If your muscles involved in the breathing process—generally those located around your ribs—are tight and stiff, they can restrict your breathing. A session in a massage chair relaxes these muscles and allows you to be able to take deeper cleansing breaths. Just a few sessions may very well improve your breathing processes.

Proper breathing is essential to many areas of your health. Doctors have known for a very long time that saturating the injured area with oxygen speeds up the healing process. Blood flows throughout the body, carrying healing oxygen with it. The greater the blood flow, the more efficient the healing process. Individuals with diabetic foot sores are an example. Because of lack of circulation and therefore lack of proper blood supply, these individuals have a difficult time healing. Smokers suffer the same healing fate... the more you smoke, the greater the constriction of the blood vessels, and the slower the healing process. Massage enhances blood flow!

- Lymph and blood flow work together to eliminate toxins from the body. When we exert our muscles, they produce a chemical known as lactic acid. Sitting in a massage chair enables the muscles to rest. While the muscles are at rest, the lymph and blood systems are better capable of removing lactic acid from the body.

- As mentioned above, oxygen and proper circulation of the blood assist the body in healing itself on the inside as well as outside. This means they will heal internal injuries such as muscle sprains as well as injuries to skin and soft tissues.

- Massage therapy can also help reduce systolic and diastolic blood pressure. Hypertension, also known as high blood pressure, affects about one-third of American adults. Simply relaxing reduces the human heart rate and therefore reduces blood pressure. Many doctors recommend that individuals learn to control their temper to keep their blood pressure from rising. One way is to count to ten. You can count ten sheep in your massage chair on your way to peaceful dreams. Massage will certainly help you relax, which may lead to lower blood pressure.

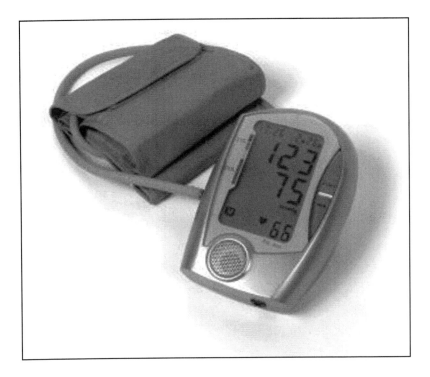

- Massage therapy can help raise your endorphin level. Our endorphins are vital to our health. They are the regulators of our bodies. It is believed that the human body produces about twenty different types of endorphins each day. Serotonin, one endorphin that the body produces, plays a major part in appetite, sleep, memory, learning, body temperature, and mood. Endorphins also help reduce pain. Massage is only one method of increasing levels of endorphins. Two others are chiropractic manipulation and exercise.

- Since massage has so very many physiological benefits, it is easy to understand why it is a great healing alternative; however, massage is also great for mental well-being. The body works through cycles. If you are tired and in constant physical pain, you can become drained emotionally. This adversely affects your mental health. If you are mentally or emotionally depleted, your body's ability to heal itself can be compromised significantly. Utilizing massage therapy will improve your physical health, which will lead to improvement in your mental health. This promotes a continuous overall sense of well-being.

Benefits of Using a Massage Chair vs. a Licensed Massage Therapist

Those who have visited a professional massage therapist know how much relief such therapy can bring. But there are some advantages of using a massage chair in your home over regular visits to a massage therapist. Here are a couple of big things to consider:

1. Cost

If you are frequenting a licensed massage therapist, you are probably paying anywhere from $60 to $150 per hour, including tips, not to mention the cost of gas and wear and tear on your car. It doesn't take a math genius to see that, over time, the cost of regular massage can be quite prohibitive. I have many, many people call me looking for a massage chair because they are shelling out so many bucks on regular massage therapy that they figure it can't be any more expensive to get a good massage chair.

Granted, a good massage chair is not cheap, but if you work the numbers, you will see that the chair pays for itself fairly quickly.

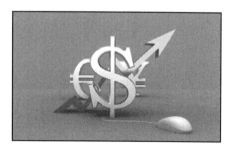

2. Convenience

Convenience may be an even bigger advantage than the cost factor! When you think about having to get dressed up, leave the comfort of your home, deal with traffic, and then come home, only to know that you will have to go through the same routine every time you want to have a massage, a massage chair right next to you sounds pretty appealing.

The chair is at your beck and call 24/7, all year long. You can use it on holidays, in the middle of the night, when you are sick, when you have no transportation, when you are in your underwear, when your hair and makeup aren't quite right, and multiple times per day. PLUS, you can reproduce what works for you with every session. Your chair delivers consistency all the time.

Chapter 2

Who Can Benefit from Owning a Massage Chair?

In Chapter 3, I discuss the physiological health benefits of massage therapy and massage chairs. What I don't discuss is who can benefit from a massage chair based on the physiological benefits.

Here is a quick list of reasons most people get a massage chair. You will most likely be able to relate to at least one of these. I might mention here that you don't have to have a condition of any sort to get a massage chair. They are just wonderful therapies that will do you a world of good whether you suffer from a condition or not. If you are pain or stress free, you can think of a massage chair as preventative therapy.

Although a massage chair does not guarantee getting rid of any condition, the conditions that involve the soft tissues of the spine have a greater chance for help from one of these chairs. The majority of the symptoms listed below are musculoskeletal in nature and thus the most common reasons for getting a massage chair.

My experience has been that if you have responded positively in any way to conservative therapy in the past for your condition(s)—chiropractic therapy, massage therapy, physical therapy, etc.—your symptoms have a fantastic chance of getting some relief from a massage chair.

1. **Back and Neck Pain** – These two symptoms are the main reasons for massage chair ownership. They are also the main reasons folks go shopping for massage chairs, as you may well be doing at this moment! Of all the things that massage chairs can do for the

body, back and neck pain relief is what they are most prominently known for.

2. **Shoulder Pain** – Shoulder pain can mean different things to different people. For example, "shoulder" to one person may mean between the shoulder blades, to another it may mean the trapezia muscles at the top of the shoulders, and yet to another it may mean the actual shoulder joint.

All massage chairs address the region between the shoulder blades (scapulae) to one degree or another, but a few also hit the tops of the shoulders. Not many chairs actually massage the outside of the shoulders (deltoid muscles) or the shoulder joint itself.

3. **Headaches** – The types of headaches that respond the best to massage chair therapy are stress-related, aka cervicogenic, headaches. These are the headaches that normally originate from muscular tissue in the neck, shoulders, and base of the skull. The user will typically have discomfort at the base of the skull and around the head in a hatlike distribution.

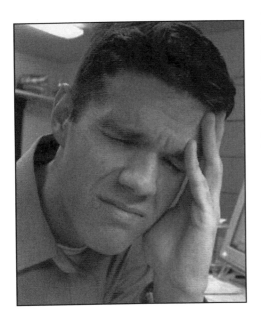

Headaches that are vascular or neurological in nature—i.e., true migraine and/or cluster headaches—will most likely not respond well to massage chair therapy. I qualify migraine headaches because a true migraine headache is actually a vascular incident related to blood circulation. Many people will claim that they have migraine headaches, speaking more to the intensity of the pain than to its origin, but that pain follows a stress-related, cervicogenic pain pattern rather than a vascular pain pattern.

4. Hip Pain – As with shoulder pain, hip pain can mean different things to different people. It can mean the thighs, the sacral area at the top of the buttocks, the butt itself, or the actual hip joint where the leg meets the pelvis.

As far as the butt muscles go (gluteals), most chairs have airbags in the seat that, at the very least, inflate against the butt muscles. Some even have rollers that extend down the length of the spine and the buttocks to the top of the hamstrings. Others have airbags that move the seat from side to side, and yet others have airbags that inflate against the outside of the thighs and massage the iliotibial band muscles.

Each feature may or may not work on the hip, however you may define it. Using the chair is the only sure way to know if the chair will do you any good. I have not seen as much symptomatic relief in this area from massage chairs as I have seen in the back and neck, so you will have to play with the chair a bit to see if it does you any good.

5. Sciatica – A typical definition of sciatica (thank you, Google!) is "pain, weakness, numbness, or tingling in the leg. It is caused by injury to or pressure on the sciatic nerve."

The actual cause of sciatica can be one of many things: herniated disc, degenerative arthritis, tumor or cyst, spinal stenosis, muscle spasm, and trauma, among other things. Massage chairs are not known to be great therapies for sciatica, but of all the causes of sciatica, a massage chair has the greatest chance of helping that caused by muscle spasm.

In practice, I remember many patients with sciatica who had corresponding spasm and tightness of the piriformis muscle(s). That is a muscle that extends across the buttocks, on each side and through which the sciatic nerve often passes. This kind of spasm is more common in women because of the changes that occur in pelvis alignment following child delivery, but men suffer from it as well. A massage chair with roller technology extending into the buttocks has the greatest chance of helping out with this form of sciatica. Chairs with seat airbags may also help, but those airbags will not have as great a chance of affecting the piriformis as rollers do.

6. **Degenerative Arthritis (aka Osteoarthritis)** – As we age, the effects of living begin to take their toll in the form of a degenerating spine. I personally played sports my life and now have the reduced range of motion and scar tissue to prove it!

The spine degenerates when spinal segments fuse together and, because of the altered movement patterns of the spine as a result of a lifetime of activity, discs thin. This type of degenerative arthritis also leads to muscle tightness and spasms.

The rollers and airbags of a massage chair will do wonders for degenerative arthritis in two ways: 1) by introducing passive motion to the spine that you ordinarily would not get during a regular day of normal activity, and 2) by reducing muscle spasms and tightness. You will find that a decrease in pain and discomfort will most likely be accompanied by an increase in range of motion...you will see that you can turn and bend further!

As a matter of fact, you may even find that the whole degenerative process slows down in your body with regular massage chair therapy.

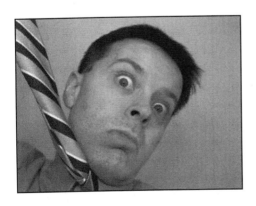

7. **Stress** – Whether or not you experience pain, I can assure you that a massage chair will bring a feeling of well-being and relaxation to your frayed body and soul. With all the activities and responsibilities you have going on during a normal day, a chair will bring a level of stress relief that you

didn't think possible. Physiologically, you may see a decrease in your blood pressure, your breathing may slow down, and sleep may more quickly settle in. This is one of the main reasons people invest in massage chairs…for the pure enjoyment of relaxation and stress relief. I promise you that the following words will come out of your mouth, in one form or another…"ooooohhhhh" and "aaaaahhhhhh!"

8. **Surprises!** – When I first began selling massage chairs, our staff and I would go to trade shows—i.e., home shows, boat shows, etc.— and hundreds of people would sit in our chairs. Invariably, we would have one or two come back after having sat in a chair and say that something interesting happened to them regarding their health. Two people who immediately come to my mind are a diabetic who hadn't had normal feeling in his legs for years who suddenly had sensation back in both legs, and a lady who had suffered from "migraines" for years who returned to our booth exclaiming that the chair had taken away her headache.

Although I would never say that a massage chair cured such-and-such a disease, I will say that very interesting things happen from time to time that just leaves me shaking my head in amazement. So don't be too surprised if you find some crazy health benefit just from sitting in a massage chair each day.

Chapter 3

8 Things You Absolutely Must Know Before You Even Consider Investing in a High-Quality Robotic Massage Chair

In the next few pages, I'm going to lay out the eight key things you **need and deserve** to have in mind before deciding what massage chair to bring into your life, what brand of massage chair to buy...and which massage chair reseller to purchase it from.

Obviously, I think that Massage-Chair-Relief.com is the best place for you to buy your new massage chair...but even if you don't decide to do business with us, you'll still learn valuable information in these pages that will make your purchase of a new massage chair as simple as possible...and will help ensure you make a wise investment that will pay you back in pain relief and comfort for years to come.

Here's What You Need to Know Before You Even Consider Buying a Robotic Massage Chair

1. What features should you look for in a massage chair?

Not so long ago a, "massage chair" was just a regular living room chair with a vibrating motor built into it. It didn't do much to massage the body or to relieve pain, but it was great if you wanted to shake up your lunch.

The point of a massage chair is to simulate the therapeutic effects of a massage therapist. If you've ever had a professional massage, you know that a talented therapist uses a number of techniques.

Whether you're buying your massage chair for comfort or to deal with a chronic pain condition such as sciatica or a painful midback, you'll want to make sure the chair has (at the very least) the following settings:

Kneading – Called *Shiatsu* by some, kneading rolls from the center of the spine outward and feels like two hands alternately rubbing your back. A kneading massage is a great way to relieve stress and give your overworked back muscles a break.

Percussion/Tapping – Have you ever seen a massage therapist "karate-chopping" someone's back? A percussive massage really gets the blood flowing and feels amazing. It's particularly good if you've been doing a lot of intense exercise.

Rolling – In my chiropractic office, I have a $2,800 table called a *roller table*. It's basically just wheels that roll up and down either side of your spine, gently moving the spinal bones and stretching your spine and muscles. Most quality massage chairs come with rolling action as standard. When you sit in one of these chairs and feel it push your spine back into position, you'll understand why it's so popular.

Full Recline – To truly get a deep tissue massage, you need to put as much of your weight onto your massage chair as possible. Unfortunately, many of the popular massage chairs out there recline only to a paltry 135 degrees. For maximum benefit, I'd recommend you get a chair that reclines 170 to 180 degrees so that you can lie down and truly enjoy your massage. (This is particularly important if you suffer from sciatica and find sitting difficult or painful.)

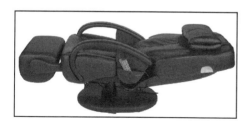

Stretch Program – Stretch programs have pretty much become the norm on most chairs nowadays. In my many years of massage chair experience, I'd have to say that the stretch program is one of the most enjoyed automatic programs by our customers. It can be very soothing. I don't really consider it a stretch program as much as I consider it a "milking" program, because it basically involves the chair back and the ottoman going up and down to "milk" the discs to keep them moving. Discs are nourished by movement of fluids in the discs. The milking action keeps the fluids in the discs moving and, thus, keeps the discs nourished.

Airbag Massage - This is truly an optional feature, but if you've ever experienced a good foot and calf massage, arm massage, or seat massage, you know how wonderful it can feel. Nowadays, chairs come with airbags that can even massage your shoulders, move your seat from side to side, work on your slumping posture, and massage your head!

Many new chairs now come with additional innovative features such as mechanical foot rollers, zero-gravity positioning, inversion, extended roller tracks down the back and into the buttocks, chromotherapy (lights on the chair body), music systems, and even head massagers! They are all pretty cool features, but you need to decide what is important to you and which features make the most sense to you. More features usually means more money...so if your pocketbook has something to say about which chair to get, you may not be able to get all the features I've listed above.

2. How durable is your chair?

Unfortunately there are many, many knockoff massage chairs being sold online...chairs that are hacked together cheaply in Chinese factories, that don't live up to their promises or do what they're meant to, and that are prone to breaking at a moment's notice.

When I was looking for **my** first massage chair, I discovered that there are two big factors to think about to make sure that you get a quality chair that will last you for years to come. They are:

How long is your chair's warranty? The longer the warranty offered by the manufacturer of the chair, the more confidence they have in their product. But don't be fooled by fly-by-night online companies who offer outrageous ten-year warranties on a $2,000 massage chair. Good luck finding your retailer or massage chair importer in six months when you have a problem with your chair! A ten-year warranty doesn't mean anything if you can't get a hold of the company that sold you the chair!! Most of the good massage chair manufacturers (such as the ones we represent) offer a rock-solid three-to-five-year limited warranty. Actually, Inada has come out with a three-year comprehensive, on-site warranty for all their chairs, while Panasonic has introduced not only a three-year parts and labor, in-home warranty on their top-tier chairs, but also two additional years of parts only. Both warranties are the best in the business.

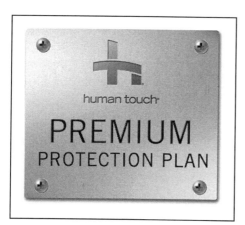

The majority of other companies offer a one-year parts and labor in-home warranty with a second year of parts and a third year of structure/frame coverage. That is pretty typical. There are a few examples of chairs that offer a two-year parts and labor in-home warranty.

Most companies will also offer extended warranty options, most of which are for one or two extra years of parts and labor in-home coverage. My experience in the industry is that these extended warranty options are a good investment.

What's the reputation of the brand? Beware of strange-sounding or rare brands. Yes, it's possible that a little-known brand has a high-quality product, but with an investment like a massage chair, you want to be safe, not sorry. In my experience, I've found Inada, Human Touch, Panasonic, Infinity, Luraco, Osaki, and Cozzia to offer higher-quality chairs backed by great warranties.

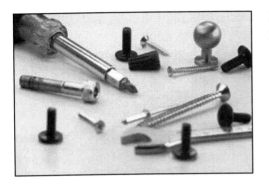

3. How easy is your chair to repair?

Even the best massage chair may eventually break down. Make sure your massage chair is built with a modular design (most are nowadays) so that it can be easily repaired...and so that you can repair it without having to send the whole chair back to the manufacturer. Not to brag, but virtually every chair we sell at Massage-Chair-Relief.com has a sturdy modular design...not to mention a reputation for durability. Be careful of warranties that, in the small print, expect you to ship the chair back to the company if you need a repair. We prefer to recommend chairs that have in-home warranties, especially during the first year.

Make sure, also, that your massage chair manufacturer has easy-to-reach customer support after the sale. If you have a problem with your chair and you call customer support, there had better be someone at the other end of the phone picking up and interacting with you about your chair. If you do decide to purchase your new massage chair from Massage-Chair-Relief.com, you can always call us if you feel like you are not being heard by the company that is providing the warranty. We can get involved and often expedite a response to your concerns.

4. What's the reputation of the reseller?

Unfortunately, there are many fly-by-night online companies out there selling massage chairs to make a quick buck. Honestly, most of the sites you see aren't really companies at all but just marketing middlemen who don't provide any real value and operate a website from their kitchen.

For such an expensive item, you'll want to make sure that your reseller has plenty of testimonials and reviews, a great reputation for customer service, and an absolute reputation for putting the customer first. My personal opinion is that they should also have a brick-and-mortar showroom where you can actually chat with a live person and try out the chairs in person.

At Massage-Chair-Relief.com, we've compiled a long list of testimonials from happy customers, and we pride ourselves on making sure all customers are ecstatic both with the product they buy and the service they receive. And of course, you can always visit our showroom to check out the chairs for yourself. You will see that we are real people, and we really do what we say we do!

5. Does the retailer have a money-back guarantee?

Buying a big item such as a massage chair online does in fact have some risk to it. What if you get the chair delivered and it doesn't fit your decor? Or what if it just isn't as comfortable or therapeutic as you were hoping? Or what if you decide that you just don't want one?

Before clicking the "order now" button or picking up the phone, make sure that your reseller offers a strong money-back guarantee… and that you don't get stuck paying the shipping costs to your home or office.

At Massage-Chair-Relief.com, we have a best-in-industry 90-day no-questions-asked money-back guarantee. If you aren't happy with your chair for **any** reason, just let us know, and we'll refund your money in full…and remember, we offer free shipping of your chair to you. Pretty much every company, including Massage Chair

Relief, will put the responsibility of return shipping on you, but we don't charge any restocking or handling fees.

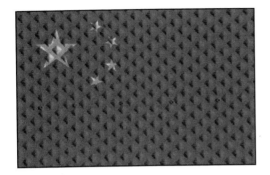

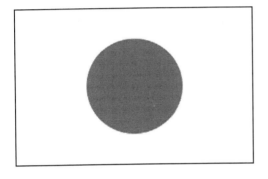

6. Chinese vs. Japanese

In all the years I've been involved in the massage chair industry, it was always commonly accepted and known that the Japanese made the best quality massage chairs. After all, Japan is the fountainhead of massage chairs, where they were invented and have been produced for over 50 years.

Manufacturing of massage chairs began in China some years ago because of lower production costs. Nowadays, the vast majority of massage chairs are being manufactured in mainland China with a few models being produced in Taiwan.

The quality of Japanese chairs has always been second to none. Inada and Panasonic, the two Japanese massage chair companies, have failure rates on their chairs of only 1% or less. Chinese chairs have a higher failure rate, some putting that rate at between 2%–5%.

Even though Chinese chairs have a higher failure rate, the chair quality has been improving over the years. Since most of the manufacturing now occurs in China, they have the capacity to hire the talent and skill for the design, engineering, and manufacturing processes. I think it is showing in the chairs that come out of China today.

Inada and Panasonic have always been Japanese companies, and their chairs have always been manufactured in Japan. Their costs and thus prices are higher because of that. Panasonic, in an effort to lower manufacturing costs, moved all their production to mainland China. However, design, engineering, and production oversight are still being done by the Japanese. Panasonic owns its own plants in China to maintain quality control.

When deciding on which chair to buy, many people want to get the best quality on the market regardless of price. If that is the approach you have, then Inada and Panasonic are the way to go.

If you have a tight budget and want a good bang for your buck, then a Chinese chair will be just fine for you...and you'll find something great for the money you have to spend.

Whatever the case, it will be good for you to know what type of shopper you are so that you can determine the perfect balance between cost, value, and quality.

7. Fitting in a massage chair

When you study massage chairs online, you may find a model that looks just perfect for you. It has all the features you want, a body styling that is cool, and a price that fits right within your budget. On paper, it is everything you want.

You order your perfect chair, get it in your home, assemble it, and then get a chance to sit in it. Within a few seconds, you realize that this chair just doesn't fit your body right. This is not uncommon, by the way.

Here are a few things to consider when checking out massage chairs to find out if it is going to be the right fit for you...

a) Body Height

Each chair model has a recommended height and weight limit. Make sure you are aware of those limits. Regarding height, some chairs do not accommodate folks over 6' very well, while others are not great for shorter frames. You can check out our comparison chart to see figures for each model we carry. Here is a link to that chart:

http://www.massage-chair-relief.com/massage-chair-comparison/

You can select any models you'd like information for and see what their height recommendations are. Though some chairs have recommended height limitations, folks that are taller or shorter than the recommendations can still find ways to make the chair work for them. I have customers who are over 6'7" tall, and there are few, if any, chairs designed for heights greater than that. But those customers have been able to adapt to the chair restrictions and still get a great massage. Their head may be too high up for the neck to get

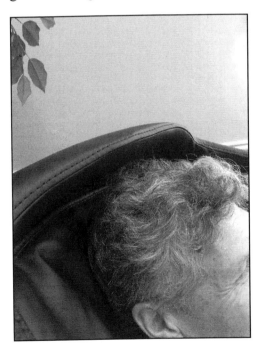

a great massage or their legs may be too long to get a comfortable seating position while getting massaged, but the user is able to work around those restrictions and make the chair work for them.

Some chairs, however, have a hard stop at the top of the chair. You can try to fit in the chair, but you will feel like one of the wicked stepsisters trying to fit Cinderella's glass slipper…it just won't work. You see, some chairs have a hard dome at the top of the chair back and thus a hard stop. There is no reasonable way for a body to fit in that chair if it is above the maximum height restriction. It just won't work.

There are also chairs that have no ottoman extension so that a tall person will not be able to get the full benefit of the leg and calf massage. His or her feet may fit in, but the knees will be up so high and so far forward that the calves may not even fit in the calf wells to get any type of calf massage at all.

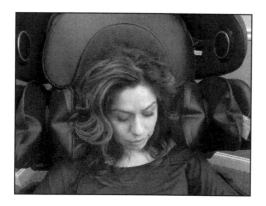

I've been focusing on the taller folks so far. What about chairs that don't work for shorter frames? I have one chair that has shoulder airbags that inflate to the front of the shoulders to pin the shoulders back and work on poor posture. Well, that chair has a minimum recommended height of 5'5". I actually took a picture of a neighbor of mine in that chair with the shoulder airbags inflated. She is only 5'0" tall, and you'll never guess where the shoulder airbags hit her. Not her shoulders, that's for sure. They inflated on her neck and chin. They didn't do anything for her except give her claustrophobia. That same chair also has waist airbags that inflated against the back of her arms rather than her waist because her torso was too short.

Needless to say, she didn't like that chair at all.

Bottom line…make sure you fit in the chair you are interested in or else you will have a chair delivered to your door that will not work at all.

b) Body Weight

Just like height, each massage chair has a recommended maximum weight limit. I've not seen a chair with a minimum recommended weight limit yet. Most chairs that are on the market have a weight limit of around 265–285 pounds. Some chairs can cater to a weight of 350 pounds and some as light as 220 pounds.

Inada actually has a motto for the weight restrictions of their chairs: "If you can fit, you can sit." In other words, if you can fit in the chair, regardless of your weight, you can sit in the chair without any weight restrictions.

Chairs have weight restrictions for a reason...the hardware of the chair may break down if the strain on the components is too great. Motors may tend to break down if the workload is too great. The structure or frame of the chair may be compromised by excessive weight.

Again, as with height, make sure you fit within the weight parameters of the chair in which you are interested. You can use the comparison chart mentioned in bullet point a) above.

c) Body Girth

You may fit fine within the recommended height and weight restrictions of the chair you want, but the shape of your body—i.e., the girth of your body—may not be a good match for the chair you are looking at.

What comes to my mind are the shoulder airbags and hip airbags that we see on a lot of chairs nowadays. For example, if you are a very broad-shouldered or broad-chested male, you may not fit well in a chair that has shoulder airbags. You see, these shoulder airbags are fitted into a hard, durable plastic housing that does not give at all. If your shoulders are so broad that you cannot fit your chest between the shoulder airbag housings on each side of the chair back, that chair will not work for you.

Also, if you have a large pelvis/hip area, you may not fit well in a chair that has hip airbags that take up a significant portion of the seat width. Be cognizant of these two things when trying to find a chair that fits you well.

d) Leg Length vs. Torso Length

I am about 5'9" tall, but I am more torso than legs. Some folks, such as my wife, are all legs. Some chairs have ottomans that don't extend very far. If you are a person with shorter legs, you may fit just fine in a chair with a restricted ottoman extension. On the other hand, if you have longer legs yet your overall height fits within a chair's specific recommendations, you may feel that your legs are cramped, as though you are sitting on an amusement park ride for kids. It just won't feel right.

You may be the perfect weight and height, but your proportions maybe different. That could be a factor in your decision-making process. I will add that this is not a huge problem for most folks, but it is something that we see from time to time that needs to be addressed or else, again, the user experience won't be optimal.

It helps so much to be able to sit in a massage chair before buying it. Size restrictions are some of the most important reasons why. If you can, please try to sit in a chair before buying it. If you can't find chairs to try out, you can always come to our showroom and experience our chairs before making a decision.

http://www.massage-chair-relief.com/out-of-state.html

8. Size of chair vs. space in your home or business

Massage chairs are getting progressively larger and more space-consuming. With arm airbags housed in armrests, larger body frames, and bigger chair backs to house larger motors and electronic components, these chairs can take up a lot of space. You will need to consider this when making a decision about a chair, especially if your residential or business space is limited.

Of course, beyond the actual dimensions of the chair itself, you will have to allot space away from the wall so that you can recline the chair back to a full extension position. So you will need to take that into consideration as well.

Some chairs now come with space-saving features such as a sliding base. With a sliding base, you can place your chair right up against any wall, and when the chair is turned on and begins a massage program, the chair body will slide forward on its base before it reclines to begin the massage. When the massage program ends, the chair will slide back on its base to its resting position right up against the wall.

I might mention here that if you get a chair that does not have a sliding base, I strongly recommend that you set the chair up a few feet away from the wall. When the chair is assembled, recline it fully and then slide the chair up against the wall in the fully reclined position. Then you will know how far away from the wall the chair should be in a resting position. This will prevent you from getting lovely holes in the wall from a reclining chair back that is too close to the wall in the first place!

The newer, larger chairs often come in more than one box. You will usually have the chair body in one box and the armrests and ottoman in another one or two boxes. The reason is that the chair packed in one box will not fit through a normal doorway. Once the chair is assembled, the same physics apply. You will not be able to get most new chairs through a normal doorway should you want to move yours from one room to another. You will have to disassemble at least one of the armrests to get it through the doorway.

One last tip when it comes to bringing a new chair into your home: if you have a hardwood floor, you might consider getting a small rug to place underneath the chair. Sometimes a chair will move a bit on the floor when it is running. That subtle slide may be an issue for a hardwood floor. I'm not saying that will happen, but it sure wouldn't hurt to put a little rug underneath the chair base to prevent any wood damage whatsoever.

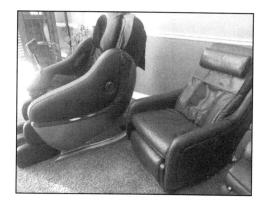

And that's really all you need to know to make a smart choice when it comes to buying a high-quality robotic massage chair that will give you many years of pain relief and increased comfort.

Of course, when you do decide that it's time to invest in a high-quality robotic massage chair, I hope that you'll visit us at Massage-Chair-Relief.com.

As a chiropractic doctor with a vested interest in the health and wellness of my patients, I've personally tested and researched chairs from every manufacturer we represent to make sure they meet my own strict standards for comfort, longevity, value, and therapeutic effectiveness.

Chapter 4

A Massage Chair for Your Business

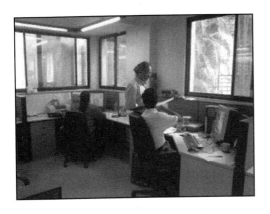

Most customers are looking for a massage chair for their home. But increasingly, we are seeing more and more businesses implementing massage chairs for their customers and/or their employees.

Here are some advantages of having a massage chair in your business:

FOR EMPLOYEES...
Increased employee loyalty
Increased individual productivity
Improved office morale
Fewer sick days
Stress relief
Improved work environment

FOR CUSTOMERS...
Increased loyalty
Positive customer experience
Improved relationship with business
Reduced anxiety
Leaves a lasting impression

You see, massage chairs can make everyone happy! I first got into the massage chair business as a chiropractor. I ordered a chair for my patients to sit in while they were waiting for treatment. It didn't take long for me to realize that the chair became part of the therapy and that patients absolutely loved it. I also found that my staff was sitting in the chair before and after work. Everyone seemed to want to get a piece of the massage chair.

In a business setting, massage chairs will give you a unique competitive advantage with both customers and employees. Many software companies are now employing massage chairs as part of an overall incentive package to attract employees.

A massage chair in your business will also motivate customers to return to sit in the chair while they are waiting for your product or service. As a matter of fact, a local tire store here in Utah uses a massage chair in their waiting room for folks waiting to have their car serviced. The owner tells me that one chair is not enough because customers are in line waiting to use the chair (he jokingly said that the customers were fighting to get into the chair before someone else did!).

I might add that a massage chair in your business will even motivate your current customers to refer new customers to you. We see this a lot with dentists who use a massage chair in their practice. Going to the dentist is, for some, a very stressful experience. A massage chair is a wonderful antidote to that anxiety. When potential patients hear about the massage chair from their friends who are current patients, the appeal is great enough that it entices many to try out the new dentist.

Some employers erroneously think that the chair will just invite staff to get lazy and sit in the chair all day long. We have not found that to be the case when a chair is used as an employee incentive tool. As a matter of fact, we have found the opposite to be true. Employees feel invigorated, refreshed, and ready to be more productive in their work.

Additionally, you will most likely find that another benefit of the massage chair is fewer workdays lost to back pain and headaches. You may find that your business productivity goes up just because of that single benefit alone.

I could go on and on discussing the benefits of having a massage chair in your business, but I'll end it here. What I'd like to discuss now are the things you should consider if you're thinking of bringing massage chairs into your business.

1. Commercial Warranty Coverage

Every massage chair comes with a warranty of some sort, but for some massage chair companies, those warranties apply only to residential use of the chair. You will need to be vigilant when deciding on a chair to know if the chair has a warranty that is applicable in commercial settings.

If you are a sole user of the chair and it sits in your office at work, then the accompanying residential-grade warranty is likely going to be fine. But if the chair is used in a situation where multiple people will get a massage throughout the day, then the commercial warranty will be needed. These types of settings would include a spa, a tire store, or a chair used in an employee lunch room. We will call this the *multi-user commercial setting (MUCS)*.

Here are three examples of the different types of warranty coverage that currently exist in the industry:

a) Inada's residential warranty does not apply to commercial settings. You would need to purchase a commercial-grade warranty for use of a chair in a MUCS.

b) Panasonic has a 1,000-hour or three-year warranty coverage for their top-tier chairs, whichever comes first. These chairs can be used in a residential or commercial setting. When the hours or time limit are used up, they are used up. They most likely would be used up more quickly in a commercial setting where many folks are sitting in the chair each day.

c) Osaki has a one-year parts and labor warranty with a second year of parts for most of their massage chairs. They will honor that warranty in either the residential or commercial setting.

Please confirm commercial warranty coverage before taking the plunge to purchase chairs for a MUCS!!

2. Synthetic Leather vs. Real Leather

Most chairs in the industry are upholstered with synthetic or faux leather. The cost of this material is less, though its durability is probably the same as real leather. The advantage of synthetic leather is the ease and lower expense of cleaning it. All you need to wipe down the synthetic is mild soapy water. For real leather, you may want to use a solution designed specifically for leather surfaces...and that will most likely cost you more.

Synthetic leather is so advanced today that it looks and feels much the same as real leather. An untrained eye would not be able to tell the difference.

3. Foot Massage?

If you get a chair that has foot massage, then you will want your employees or customers to take their shoes off. Some folks are quite uncomfortable doing that and will not sit in a massage chair to avoid taking their shoes off. And you certainly don't want people wearing shoes when they sit in your chairs because the coarseness of the shoe materials, especially the soles, will wear down the linen that is customarily used in the foot massage mechanism.

You can get massage chair models that don't have foot massagers but still have calf-massaging technology. With these chairs, as I learned in my chiropractic practice, people can leave their shoes on and not have to deal with any embarrassment that might accompany taking off shoes.

If you do get a chair that incorporates a foot-massaging mechanism, you might consider having a basket of little slip-on socks next to the chair to cover the employees' or customers' feet. This is convenient for the user as well as the business by protecting the footwells from any funky foot diseases. I use socks in our showroom for that very purpose.

4. Ease of Use

You will want a chair that is so easy to use that by simply pushing one or two buttons, your user is in massage chair heaven. Some chairs come with the need to push multiple buttons to get set up: one for reclining the chair back, one for raising the ottoman, one for turning on the chair, one or more for selecting massage functions, etc.

You will most likely want to get a chair that requires only one or two buttons to get the chair somewhat reclined and a program selected. The more automated and preset the massage, the easier it is for the user to get started and for someone to teach the user how to get started.

It would also help to have a chair that automatically returns to the "parked" position either when the program is finished or when the power button is pressed to turn off the massage. You don't want to have folks trying to figure out how to get out of a chair, which can be frustrating to new users. Remember that most folks have never sat in a massage chair before, let alone the particular model that you have purchased for your business, and there is a learning curve. Make that curve as short and sweet as possible.

QUICK TIP: Create a simple one-page "Quick-Start Guide" that a new chair user can follow to get started without any assistance from a live person. This can be in the form of a laminated card or sheet that easily demonstrates how to get the chair started and how to end the session. This will save you from having to use a staff member to train folks how to use the chair.

5. Big and Small

You undoubtedly will have customers or employees who are short, tall, wide, or thin, and all variations in between. When considering a chair for a business setting, one thing to think about is getting a chair that will accommodate the greatest number of body types. As noted before, some chairs have a height limit of 5'11" or 6'0" tall; some are made for people no shorter than 5'5" tall; and yet others have shoulder airbags that would not fit a broad-chested or broad-shouldered individual.

You will need to take these things into consideration when picking out a chair for your business. Each chair has specs to guide you. You will probably not find one chair that fits everyone, but you can find a chair that caters to the greatest spread of body sizes in your business.

6. Massage Intensity

When I first bought a massage chair for my patients, I thought every-one would love it. Of course, most people did, but there were a few who thought that the airbags and/or rollers were too intense. It made for an uncomfortable experience for some. Over time, I learned that there were chairs with airbag intensity adjustments and roller inten-sity adjustments.

Pretty much all massage chairs on the market today have airbag intensity adjustments, but only relatively few have a roller intensity adjustment feature. You can adjust the speed of the rollers in most chairs, which mimics a more intense massage experience, but the 3D roller innovation is now becoming quite popular. With this technology, you can move the rollers forward and backward to increase or decrease the degree to which the rollers dig into the spinal musculature. This is the most advanced way to change the intensity of the roller massage in massage chairs today.

Not all bodies are alike, with some people being hypersensitive and others who would have you hit their back with a sledgehammer to get the deepest massage possible! Getting 3D roller technology will cater to most everyone. It would be nice, too, if that feature was easy to access on the remote so that the user can adjust it without too much difficulty.

7. A Revenue Generator

Some businesses may want to charge customers a small fee to use their massage chair(s). This isn't uncommon in a health spa or a chiropractor's office. This turns your new massage chair into a profit center and revenue generator. Not a bad idea if this model fits your business.

8. A Business Expense

Related to our discussion in #7 of using a massage chair as a revenue generator, you can certainly consider the purchase of a massage chair as a business expense for tax purposes. Of course, I would defer any discussion of business expenses and tax write-offs to your CFO or accountant to be sure. But it is something that I get asked a lot about in this business.

A massage chair is a wonderful tool to use in your business. It can be a customer retention magnet, an employee perk, an in-office therapy, a stress manager, a pain reliever, a morale booster, a revenue generator, a treatment prep, and a loyalty booster. You may have your own ideas on how to use this amazing tool in your business.... Let your imagination run wild!

Chapter 5

Refurbished and Used Massage Chairs...Buyer Beware!

With the high price of a new massage chair, it is not uncommon for people to look for refurbished or used units. At first glance, it doesn't sound like a bad idea, but I think there are some things you need to consider before taking the plunge with a used or refurbished chair.

USED

1. Do you want your massage chair to have a warranty? Most new chairs have anywhere from one- to three-year parts and labor in-home warranty along with some parts, structure, and frame coverage after that. Used massage chairs, unless sold by an authorized dealer—i.e., a floor model or returned chair—do not come with a transferred warranty. If you run across a private sale and the seller is touting an existing warranty that will transfer to the new owner... be very wary! To really make sure, ask for the make and model of the chair along with the serial number and name of the buyer so that you can call the massage chair company and verify when the chair was bought, if the warranty can even be transferred, if there is any warranty remaining, and, if so, how much time is left and what is covered.

It is a really, really good idea to always find out what the make and model of the chair are and call the massage chair company to find out what little details might need to be known before purchase.

If a warranty on a used chair is not important to you, then ignore what I just told you.

2. Make sure the chair you are buying was built or imported by a well-known company. Should something go wrong with the chair while you own it, it is great to know that you can get parts for the chair, with or without any warranty coverage. If you are not sure about a chair company, feel free to give me a call, and I can let you know.

3. If the used chair you are looking at is a discontinued model by the maker or importer of the chair, check with the company to make sure that parts are still available. I will discuss this topic more in the "Refurbished" section below.

REFURBISHED

You can find refurbished chairs, but the single biggest problem with them is whether or not the company that made or imported the chair still makes it, let alone if the company even still exists! If the chair has been discontinued, you may have great difficulty getting parts for it.

I had two experiences with this pertaining to the HT-1650 by Human Touch. The chair was a popular seller before it was discontinued and replaced with the HT-9500. For two clients of mine, the chair broke down, and when the customers called Human Touch to get a part for the chair's repair, they were told that the parts they needed were no longer available. If they wanted to keep a semblance of the chair, they would have to purchase the new HT-9500. Fortunately, Human Touch had a generous purchase plan for customers who could no longer get their HT-1650 serviced. But not all companies have that available. And, even still, the customer will have to spend some significant dollars to get the replacement chair.

The warranty issue also applies to a refurbished chair, although most refurbished chairs come with a minimal warranty, i.e., 90 days or so. Plus, extended warranties are usually not available on refurbished chairs.

So the long and short of what I am saying is…if you are getting a refurbished chair, as I mentioned regarding used chairs, make sure that the parts are still available from the massage chair company. Call the company and figure out what is available and what problems you may run into down the road.

Buying new is always the best way to go when considering a massage chair (or any electronic device, for that matter) because you will always get a factory warranty to rely on should you ever have a problem with the chair. The saying "you get what you pay for" is no truer than it is in the massage chair market.

Having said that, I know of quite a few folks who bought a used chair, even a no-name brand chair, and were very happy with it. The risk of no warranty is outweighed by the good deal they got in the transaction. Some used chairs are priced so low that even if the chair broke down and could not be repaired, the buyer still felt that it was worth the risk. You will need to consider what works best for you. But as the title of this chapter says, buyer beware!!

Hope this helps!! Be careful out there.

Chapter 6

Is It Safe for Children to Use Massage Chairs?

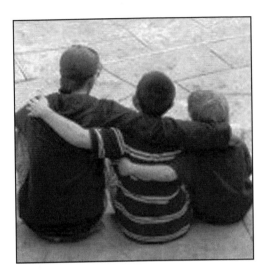

I have had massage chairs either in my clinic or in my showroom for well over ten years, and I can say without reservation that I have never seen a child not enjoy them! And I have had literally hundreds of kids sit on our chairs over those years and have never seen or heard a child complain about the massage being delivered by a chair. Not only is it a fun thing to sit on, what with the remote controls and such, but the kids actually love the feeling of the therapy.

Well, that is my experience in my showroom. If I didn't know anything other than that, I would positively and absolutely say that kids and massage chairs are a match made in heaven. There are no studies showing if massage chairs are good for kids. But what does the literature say about children and massage therapy in general? Is there something that might suggest that massage is contraindicated for children? Here are some interesting points about children and massage therapy:

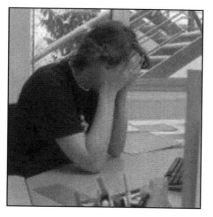

1. **Kids have stress**, just like their folks, but they don't always manifest that stress in quite the same way that we do. We all know massage is a perfect musculoskeletal antidote for stress and anxiety, so a massage chair is the perfect therapy for your kids to relieve any stress they may be experiencing. Just because they don't exhibit the same symptoms of stress as an adult does not mean they don't feel it significantly and deeply. It also doesn't mean they wouldn't benefit from a session in a massage chair.

Constant stress in children and adults results in elevated cortisol, which can damage immune cells, thus weakening the immune system. Massage chairs can relieve stress and in turn give the immune system a break.

Divorce, school, friends, etc. can be contributors to your child's stress. A massage chair can actually become a source of therapy for your children as well as for you. The kids might think it's a big toy, but they are getting actual therapeutic benefit when they sit in the chair and use it.

If your child struggles with other medical conditions that are exacerbated by stress—e.g., diabetes, stress-induced asthma, and autoimmune diseases—the massage from a chair may also help with those symptoms as well.

2. **Nationwide Children's Hospital** actually has a staff of full-time licensed massage therapists because of the profound healing effects of massage. I am aware of a hospital in Canada that, at the time of this writing, had 30 massage chairs available to patients and their families.

What's interesting about Nationwide Children's Hospital is that they offer massage to patients with the following conditions:

Cardiopulmonary

Cystic fibrosis

Heart/lung transplant

ECMO (Extracorporeal Membrane Oxygenation)

Asthma

BPD (Broncho-Pulmonary Dysplasia)

Oncology

Childhood cancers

Bone marrow transplant

Limb salvage

Hematology

Sickle cell disease

Bleeding disorders

Neurology

Migraine headaches

Seizures

Spinal cord injuries

Head injuries

Eating Disorders

Anorexia nervosa

Bulimia

Rumination

Failure to thrive

Trauma

Traumatic brain injuries

Spinal cord injuries

Burns

Orthopedic conditions

Chemical Dependency

To be honest, I was surprised by the number and severity of the conditions in a children's hospital which massage therapy can address. It was a pretty impressive list.

3. Though the research on this is sparse yet promising, many massage therapists claim that massage helps **children with autism**. Some of these very limited studies "showed that massage therapy did provide significant benefits in the areas of social communication, adaptive behavior, and sensory profile" (www.autismdailynewscast.com). Autism is becoming one of the most commonly diagnosed

conditions in America. If massage can help and, extrapolating from that assumption, massage chairs can offer anything similar, they could be a great therapy for autistic kids.

Other therapists report that children with autistic symptoms show increased relaxation during activities, more so than with any other relaxation method.

4. In a 2003 study of the *Journal of the Canadian Academy of Child and Adolescent Psychiatry*, massage and exercise therapy were found to help **ADHD kids**. It was reported in the study that after six weeks, the kids who were in the massage group exhibited better anger control, improvement in mood, more restful sleep, an improvement in social functioning in two out of three participants, and improvement in focusing at school. It was also found that parents felt as if they could contribute more to their child's well-being after having been disappointed with the traditional medical approach.

Like the studies done in #3 above, the sample size was too small to make definitive conclusions, but all of these studies led researchers to believe that the results merited longer-term studies on these subjects.

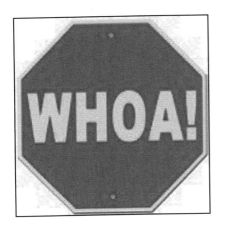

Contraindications for Massage Therapy in Kids

Although massage therapy is obviously a great therapy for children, there are also some contraindications of massage, and from what I have read, they are much the same as those for adults. If you have any of the following conditions, please consult with a doctor to confirm that massage would be OK for your child.

I might just add that although diabetes is on the list, my type 1 diabetic 27-year-old daughter uses massage chairs regularly without any negative consequences.

Also, when cancer is mentioned, my training as a chiropractor taught us not to apply massage to a part of the body that has a cancerous tumor. However, if you have cancer in a body location distant from the areas that the chair will apply massage therapy to, you are probably OK to use the chair. I have a recent customer who has liver cancer, and his oncologist said it was fine to use a massage chair. So, again, consult with your doc if you have any of these conditions or if you have any other concerns about using a massage chair with your medical condition.

Contraindications can be local or complete. *Local* means that in certain situations, massage may still be indicated depending on the locale of the condition. *Complete* generally means that it is definitely a no-no to apply massage therapy. Again, if you are not sure or are concerned about using a massage chair in any of these situations, consult with your doctor. Here is the list (taken from http://massage.ca/contraindictionscautions.html):

Local Contraindications:

Acute inflammation

Broken bone/over a nonconsolidating fracture

Recent surgery

Inflammation of the skin

Varicosities (varicose veins) over sites with deep vein thrombosis

Local contagious conditions

Blood clots

Open wound or sore

Local irritable skin conditions

Undiagnosed lump

Acute lesion

Malignancy/active cancer

Skin infection

Tumor

Acute flare-up of rheumatoid arthritis

Recent burn

Phlebitis (inflammation of a vein)

Phlebothrombosis (blood clots in the veins)

Arteritis (inflammation of the arteries)

Complete Contraindications:

Burns (severe)
Infectious disease
Anaphylaxis (life-threatening allergic reaction)
Appendicitis (painful inflamed appendix)
Cerebrocardiovascular accident (stroke)
Insulin shock or diabetic coma
Epileptic seizure (convulsions)

Myocardial infarction (heart attack)

Pneumothorax (air or gas within the chest cavity around the lung)

Atelectasis (a collapsed portion of the lung that does not contain air)

Severe asthmatic attack

Syncope (fainting or loss of consciousness)

Acute pneumonia

Advanced kidney failure, respiratory failure, or liver failure (a very modified treatment may be possible with medical consent)

Diabetic complications such as gangrene, advanced heart or kidney disease, or very unstable high blood pressure

Eclampsia (a severe form {life-threatening} of pregnancy-induced hypertension resulting in seizures)

Hemophilia severe type (a hereditary bleeding disorder)

Hemorrhage (involves rapid and uncontrollable loss of blood)

Arthrosclerosis (severe forms of stiffening or hardening of the joints

Hypertension (unstable) (conditions that are not stable, i.e., post-stroke or heart attack)

Medical shock (a life-threatening medical emergency and one of the leading causes of death for critically ill people; the body reacts and produces insufficient blood flow to reach the body tissues)

Fever above 38.5 degrees C or 101.5 F (significant)

Some highly metastatic cancers (diagnosed not to be terminal)

Systemic contagious or infectious conditions

This list is from a website for massage therapists. Of course, a massage chair is different from the actual hands of a massage therapist, so some of these conditions may not necessarily be subject to the same caution as would be a massage therapist. Again, if you are concerned or in doubt, consult with your physician.

I hope this article puts your mind at ease about whether you child can use your new massage chair or not. Of course, if you don't want your little ones in your chair at all...just put it in your bedroom and you won't have to worry about any of the above-mentioned studies or contraindications! In a lot of cases with kids, I'd be more concerned about the health of the massage chair than the health of the kids. The kids will be fine…I'm not always so sure about the chairs, though!

Dr. Alan Weidner

www.massage-chair-relief.com

REFERENCES:

http://www.massagetherapy.com/articles/index.php/article_id/470/Children-and-Massage

http://www.nationwidechildrens.org/massage-therapy

http://www.autismdailynewscast.com/massage-therapy-for-children-with-autism-requires-further-research/3612/janetmeydam/

http://www.growingupeasier.org/index.php?main_page=page&id=160&chapter=3

http://www.ncbi.nlm.nih.gov/pmc/articles/PMC2538473/

http://www.amtamassage.org/infocenter/adhd.html

http://massage.ca/contraindictionscautions.html

Chapter 7

Massage Chairs and Pregnancy

Since my days in chiropractic practice up to my current involvement in the **massage chair** marketplace, I have often been asked questions about whether massage is safe during pregnancy. In addition, people wonder whether chiropractic adjustments, licensed massage therapy, and use of massage chairs are recommended for pregnant women.

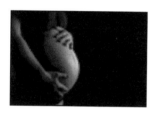

Massage Chairs and Pregnancy

Are massage chairs safe during pregnancy? My answer is the same as for all situations, and that is yes. Of course, if there are unique concerns about the baby's or your health, it is prudent to check with your physician before embarking on a program of massage therapy.

In my practice through the years, I have treated many pregnant women at all stages from the beginning to the last trimester. Naturally, there may be some tweaking of a massage regimen in the last few months because of the body's physical changes. There never have been any problems.

With all that is going on in a woman's body during pregnancy, massage has wonderful benefits during the entire nine months. For years, I have found that hands-on and manual massage are of great help to pregnant women. Since I have been involved in the massage chair industry, I have discovered no difference in the benefits of robotic massage therapy in a chair.

There is a pretty long list of health issues that can come up during pregnancy. Some of these are back and neck pain with headaches, muscle spasms, difficulty breathing, poor circulation, insomnia, reduced mobility, and strained posture. Along with any other complaints you may have, even a few of the issues on this list can make your life miserable.

A massage chair is useful to help with all of these issues:

1. *Aches and pains, muscle spasm* – Your body will experience strain on your muscles as the baby grows. This can result in pain anywhere. Your best bet is to relax your muscles. Your massage chair not only relaxes your muscles but also helps flush toxins out that have settled there and can cause pain. When your muscles relax, pain and muscle spasm subside.

I'm sure you have heard of endorphins, nature's answer to pain-killers. They are released into your bloodstream as you enjoy your massage chair. This also helps reduce those aches and pains in your body.

2. *Poor circulation with swelling* – Calf and foot massage features in massage chairs compress the legs, which helps the lymph and blood circulate better. Edema (swelling) will be reduced and toxins (discussed above) flushed from the body more efficiently.

3. *Poor posture (postural stress)* – Any pregnant woman knows about this health issue. You have this mass sticking out from your middle that throws you off-kilter. Your posture suffers. Maybe you started out your pregnancy with poor posture as well. The added strain on your muscles from postural stress often produces aches and pains.

You will find, as most folks do, that your posture improves after a massage chair session. You will stand straighter because the massage chair will work your muscles.

4. *Reduced mobility* – With forty pounds of baby, fluids, and tissue added to your body, you can't move as easily. Your joints don't seem to cooperate when you try to turn. Your massage chair sessions will amaze you as you check yourself afterwards. You will be able to turn far more easily than before.

5. *Headaches, neck and back pain* – All of the above benefits to posture, muscles, etc., will aid in reducing any pain no matter where it is located.

6. *Difficulty with breathing* – How in the world are you supposed to breathe deeply with that precious cargo pressing in on you? Actually, aside from the obvious, most pregnant women unconsciously develop a slouch. Your posture will be dramatically improved by the roller action over the middle of your back. In addition to your relaxed muscles, you will have better posture and ability to breathe more deeply. Improved sleep can result as well.

7. *Insomnia (sleeping problems)* – Countless people have told me how surprised they were to find that, after their massage chair sessions, they slept better. Your nerves relax as well as your muscles. While trying to sleep a month before you are due can be a challenge with any therapy you are involved in, the relaxation alone from your massage chair will undoubtedly help you get a better night's sleep.

With this information, your mind should be at ease about using your massage chair while pregnant.

Chapter 8

Paying for a Massage Chair

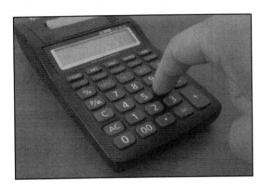

Of course, credit cards, cash, and checks are the most popular way that customers pay for a massage chair, but there are a few other options for getting a chair in your home or business:

a) **Health Savings Accounts (HSAs)** – This is a savings account that some insurance companies offer to customers into which you (and hopefully your employer) put money each year to use toward meeting your deductible and co-pays. It also can be used for buying other health-related products and services that your insurance may not pay for at all. For example, I have an insurance plan that does not cover eyeglasses, yet I can use my HSA account to pay for any eyewear or optometry costs. I just use a debit card that is issued to me by the HSA administrators.

Many HSA plans will allow for the purchase of a massage chair. You will need to contact your HSA account administrator to see if they will pay for it and what their protocol is for getting reimbursed for your expenditure or for paying it outright.

b) **Financing** – I can't speak for other online retailers, but we at Massage-Chair-Relief.com offer third-party financing options for our customers. We actually have two options: i) PayPal's Bill Me Later program, which offers a six months no payment/no interest financing,

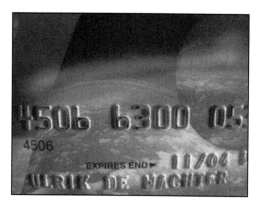

and ii) GE Capital, which offers six- or twelve-month 0% interest/minimum payment financing plans. A few times a year, GE Capital lowers its merchant processing fees so we can offer an 18-month financing plan, too.

c) **Insurance reimbursement** – I will be honest with you...since 2005, when I first started in the massage chair business, I have seen only a handful of customers who received insurance reimbursement for their massage chair purchase. I have never heard of a bill submitted for a massage chair to an insurance company getting paid. That doesn't mean that it can't happen...I just haven't seen it. Contact your insurance company to find out what you would need to do to get them to cover some or all of the cost of your chair.

You May Already Be Paying for a Massage Chair Without Even

Knowing It!

Massage chairs can cost anywhere from $1,500 to $8,000 for a name-brand chair. It sounds like a lot of money, but let's do a breakdown of that cost and what you may be already spending for musculo-skeletal complaints at doctors', physical therapists', and/or massage therapists' offices. You might be surprised how affordable a massage chair really can be.

CALCULATION #1

Let's assume that you get a massage two times per month and a chiropractic or physical therapy visit one time per month. Let's also assume that your massage costs you $80 per visit and your chiropractic visit costs you the same. So we are using a conservative estimate of $240 spent per month. This does not take into consideration the cost of gas traveling to your appointments, which we'll conservatively estimate at $10 per month, and the cost of your time to do the same. It's hard to put a price on your time, so we won't add that to the equation.

I have also not entered the cost of pain medications into this equation. Who knows how much we spend each year on pain medications, creams, orthopedic supports, new beds, pillows, and even surgeries to take care of our pain and discomfort in addition to the doctor and therapist visits? You can see how the costs can mount over the course of 52 weeks. And I might mention here that these potentially real costs are for *only one person!* Only you know how many people are in pain and paying for relief in your home throughout the year.

CALCULATION #2
Now, let's assume that you are buying a chair that costs $4,000, which is a middle-of-the-road massage chair. As I mentioned above, a massage chair could cost anywhere from $1,500 to $8,000, but at the time of this writing, our most popular chair is priced at $3,995.

THE FINAL TALLY
$250 per month x 12 months = $3,000 per year spent on doctors and therapists.

$3,995 / $250 spent per month = 16 months to pay off the chair.

So over the course of 16 months, not only are you paying for a beautiful massage chair, but you are also getting therapy 24/7, 365 days a year, not to mention pain relief. You have your own in-house massage therapist. You can't even quantify that benefit in dollars and cents.

Do you see now how affordable a massage chair really can be? In these terms, you would be considered a fiscally responsible genius to get a massage chair in your home ASAP! Oh, and don't forget that the chair can be used by everyone in the house...not just you. So for some of your family members, the costs I have discussed may be increased by some multiple of what I have shown above in calculation #1.

A massage chair just makes sense!

Chapter 9

So You Bought a Massage Chair... Now What?

Once you have purchased a massage chair, there are a few things you might want to consider in order to optimize your investment:

1. Although your massage chair was made to function without any maintenance, I would recommend cleaning the upholstery once in a while (weekly? monthly?). For synthetic leather chairs, simply using mild soapy water will do the trick. If you get a true leather upholstered chair, you might use a leather cleaner and even a leather moisturizer to help keep the leather clean and healthy.

Any areas of your chair where there is a linen covering—i.e., arms, legs, and neck—you can also use the mild soapy water to clean them. Oil, dust, and sand can get into this material and erode it over time.

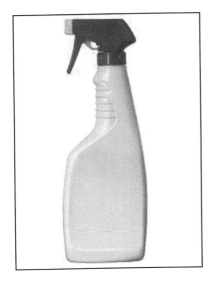

I would also strongly recommend vacuuming out the footwells and the crevice between the seat and the chair back to get sand and other accumulated junk out of there. You'll be surprised how much stuff deposits in these corners of the chair even if you just wear socks or bare feet in the chair.

2. Some chair companies require that you fill out a warranty card

and mail it back to the manufacturer. In those cases, make sure you do that to activate your warranty. Some chairs don't require any registration at all, but you may be asked to present a copy of your receipt when calling in for any warranty support. You should have received a copy of your receipt from the retailer at the time of purchase. Should you not have that copy, your retailer should be able to supply you with a copy upon request.

By the way, you should know that very few massage chair companies, if any, will transfer the chair's warranty should you choose to sell it while you still have some of the warranty left. The buyer of your chair will not have any warranty coverage. This is also important to know if you are a shopper of a used chair. You will most likely not have any warranty coverage on the chair.

3. Keep the owner's manual! You may need it for personal reference at some future time, but you may also want to keep it in case you sell the chair to a new owner. The new owners would certainly appreciate a copy of the owner's manual.

4. You might also want to keep the original packaging of the chair, especially during the money-back guarantee period of your new chair. The cost of shipping massage chairs is quite high…and that is in the original packaging. If you do not have that packaging material, your cost of shipping could go through the roof!

Keeping the packaging will also make it easier for you to transport the chair if you choose to sell it later on. However, the packaging for these chairs takes up a lot of space. If you don't have the space, then you can get rid of the material after the money-back guarantee has expired…and worry about shipping if and when the time comes for you to sell it.

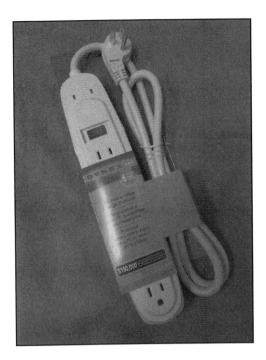

5. *Get a surge protector!!!* I recently spoke with the president of Inada USA about their failure rate. He said that for chairs that arrive at the new owner's home, the failure rate is virtually zero. If something goes wrong with the chair after it arrives at its destination, the cause is almost always electrical incidents. Surge protectors will prevent many chair breakdowns. Getting one is the single most important thing you can do for your chair once it is in your home.

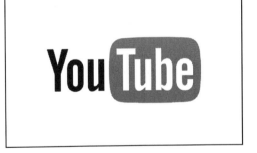

6. I would recommend tapping into any videos we have produced for your chair model on our YouTube channel to get you familiar with some of the functions and features of your new chair. Of course, we don't have videos for every massage chair, but we do for the most popular models on the market. These videos have been made to educate new and potential users of a massage chair. You can visit our YouTube channel here:

http://www.youtube.com/massagechairrelief/

7. Tell others about how wonderful your new massage chair is! I am of the firm opinion that every home and business needs a massage chair for all the health reasons mentioned in chapters 1 and 2. But I can't educate everyone about them. That is where you come in. Please help me spread the word about massage chairs and how amazing they really are. It is said that at least 25% of all homes in Japan have a massage chair. In the USA, that percentage is closer to 1% or less. Lots of work to do…let's get on it!

Chapter 10

"Why on Earth Would I Get My Massage Chair from Massage Chair Relief?"

There are plenty of massage chair retailers in the world, and making the crucial decision of whom to go with is a big one. This book has been written to help you make the right decision about a massage chair, but what information can I give you to help you make the right decision about which retailer to use? Of course, I'd love for you to invest in your new massage chair from Massage Chair Relief, but you may find something else in another store.

I'd like to make a case for our store and company if you don't mind (a bit of a sales pitch coming up!). Here are the reasons why I think that you would be best served by getting your massage chair from Massage Chair Relief:

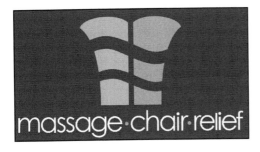

Only Store of Its Kind in the Country!

Even though we have been selling massage chairs online and offline since 2005, I actually began with massage chairs in my chiropractic clinic a couple of years before that. It all began with an old HT-125 from Human Touch that I purchased for patients to sit in while they were waiting for treatment. Our patients were so impressed with the chairs that they began to ask where they could get one. That started a path that led to where we are today, which is the premier massage chair retailer in the country.

Our showroom is the only one of its kind in the country; we have all the major name brands represented under one roof...a rarity in this industry. After I sold my practice in 2008, we immediately opened the showroom to display our chairs, and it has become the destination of choice for serious massage chair shoppers.

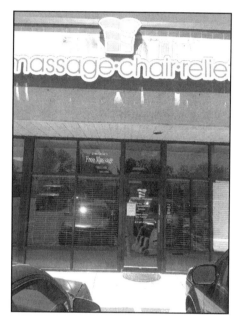

90-Day Money-Back Guarantee

I am very proud of this policy. We give you 90 days from the date of purchase to decide if you want your chair or not. There is no rush. I understand that many of the chairs are purchased sight unseen. When the chair arrives by delivery truck, it may not end up being what you expected. Well, give it a try for 90 days, and if for any reason whatsoever you don't like it or want it, you can return it.

Did you know, in fact, that every other retailer has a 30-day money-back guarantee from the time of purchase. If you think about it, your chair won't even arrive for a week or two or even three after that. That gives you very, very little time to get to know your chair and really get into it. You pretty much have to decide within a week or two if it is the right match.

Why rush? Take your time. If you feel rushed, you may make a poor decision about whether you should keep the chair or not and come to regret your decision. With 90 days, you have ample time to play with it, let your family enjoy it, see what it can do for you, overcome some of your new-chair soreness, and comfortably decide if it is right for you.

Here is something else that's pretty cool about our 90-day return policy: I don't charge handling or restocking fees! That's right... no 20%, 30%, or even 40% restocking fees. You will get your full purchase price back, less the credit card fees charged to us by your credit card company at the time of purchase (only 3%–3.5%).

Remember, it's a "no questions asked" return policy. You can return it for any reason whatsoever. All you have to pay for is the return shipping.

Out-of-Stater Program

Even though we didn't realize it at the time of our grand opening, our store was the only one in the country that housed a sampling of every major name-brand massage chair in the country. I started to have customers visit us from California, Nevada, Idaho, and Wyoming. Then we started getting folks wanting to come to our showroom when they were on a layover at the airport en route to another destination.

Then we actually had a customer fly out just to see us!! It was then that I truly grasped the uniqueness of our situation. I came up with the Out-of-Stater program as an official way to invite serious massage chair shoppers out to Utah to try out the chairs. So many people had so many questions about which chair was the right one for them...but none were able to find a place where they could try them all out under one roof.

The essence of our program is this:

You fly out to Utah at your expense, and we will take care of the rest. We pick you up at the airport, drive you to the showroom, help you select the perfect massage chair for you, take you out to lunch (at our expense!), and then drive you back to the airport for your return flight.

If you decide on a chair that is under $5,000, I will take $300 off the price of the chair to pay for all or some of the cost of your flight. If you purchase a chair that is priced over $5,000, I will take $500 off the price of the chair to that same end.

You conceivably could come to Utah, try out the chairs, get the perfect chair for you, and then return to your home state without any cost to you at all! Not a bad idea, eh? Well, it has worked for a large number of massage chair customers. It can work for you, too.

Here is a link to the page on our site that gives the details of the Out-of-Stater program:

http://www.massage-chair-relief.com/out-of-state.html

Best Price Guarantee

Since we are on the topic of guarantees, I thought this might be the right time to mention our Best Price Guarantee. If you find the chair you want anywhere else on the web or in a brick-and-mortar store for less than what we charge, I will match that price and, in some cases, even beat it! I never want to lose a chair on price alone. You see, we really shine in our customer service after the sale (read some of our reviews for proof of that). We can't give you service if we lose your business on price. I'll talk about our customer service next (this is where we really shine)…

On-Demand Customer Service

I love the term *on-demand* that the cable companies use to describe the availability of movies and shows on TV. We work hard for that to be our mantra at Massage Chair Relief. I always tell my customers that I'm as easy to reach after the sale as I am before the sale. I take pride in that. There is no hiding on our part....We will always be accessible to you should you ever have a question or concern.

There are a number of ways that you can reach us:

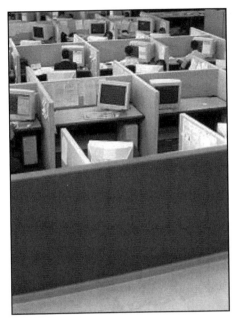

a) *Phone* – Our toll-free number is 888-259-5380, and our showroom number is 801-417-8240. I always make sure that the calls are forwarded to my phone or someone else's phone after regular business hours so that you can reach someone anytime. It is very important to me that your voice is heard.

b) *E-mail* – You can always send me an e-mail at alan@massage-chair-relief.com. I try to get to e-mails within a few hours of getting them. Some require more thoughtful answers and may take me a little longer to write, but most of the time, I can get back to you within the hour.

c) *Chat* – You can always go online to our site and use the chat feature. If no one can speak to you at that moment, leave your message and we'll get back to you as soon as possible.

We don't ever want you to feel like you are being avoided or that you are not important to us.

Make-A-Wish Foundation

This is a project that has been near and dear to my heart since my chiropractic days in clinic. We sponsored a Make-A-Wish

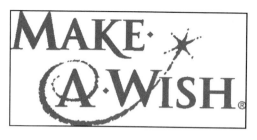

child many years ago, and the whole experience literally changed my life. I went on a tour at the local Make-A-Wish office building here in Murray, Utah, and wept like a baby as I read testimonial after testimonial of Wish Kids and realized what these kids were going through and what this organization was doing to help them through.

Our first Wish Child wanted to go to Disney World (a lot of the kids want to go there!). Our patients helped us raise enough money to see this dear little girl realize her dream. That was pretty cool…but what was *really* cool was to see her after she returned. Her mother brought her to the clinic and introduced us to her. This little gal, who couldn't talk, was so lively and cheerful. You could see the joy in her eyes and in the way she interacted with us from her wheelchair. Her mom said that she was docile and terribly introverted before the Disney World trip. It had changed her. Her mother was thrilled, and this little girl was radiating so much amazing beauty. Our whole office was so moved by the experience.

To make a long story even longer, we have carried over our commitment to granting kids their wishes at Massage Chair Relief. A portion of every massage chair we sell is donated to the Make-A-Wish Foundation on behalf of a Wish Child. You can visit the page on our site or our company page on the Make-A-Wish site to see what our goal is, who our Wish Child is, and how far along we are to reaching our goal. I'd like to encourage you to donate to this amazing project even if you decide not to use us as your massage chair retailer.

http://www.massage-chair-relief.com/make-a-wish.html

http://friends.wish.org/042-000/page/Alan-Weidner/Massage-Chair-Relief-Grants-Wishes!.htm

Extensive Video and Article Library

Massage Chair Relief has the ultimate learning center, making it your one-stop shop for research. Any topic that you want to study as you decide which chair is right for you can be found in either our article library or on our YouTube channel.

When I first got into the massage chair business back in 2005, one of my greatest desires was to create the ultimate resource for massage chair buyers. I knew that it was hard to find chairs to sit in and experience firsthand, so I figured the next best thing was to put out as much information as possible on the Internet so that everyone could have access to material that would assist in making the right choice. Of course, there is nothing like sitting in an actual massage chair, but for many people, that is next to impossible without traveling great distances.

I started writing articles right from the beginning of our business and began making videos in 2009 for our YouTube channel. Both of these resources have become among the most read and viewed media in the industry.

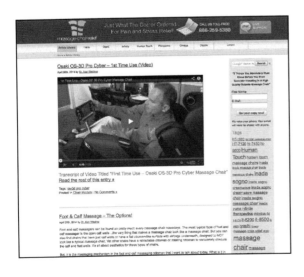

A. Article Library

This resource is full of articles (hundreds upon hundreds!) that address pretty much any and every topic about massage chairs and the industry. You can read reviews of one particular chair, comparative reviews of two chairs, articles about warranties and white glove service, and virtually any feature a massage chair can have. I've also put in the database e-mails from customers along with my responses, news updates, chair updates, and so much more.

You could literally spend an entire day sifting through the articles, finding info that will help you make your massage chair choice.

I even made a video tutorial for one of our YouTube playlists that shows you how to access the huge database of articles on www.massage-chair-relief.com. There are essentially three ways to find those articles:

i) search field on the home page (below the fold),

ii) search field on any page of the actual article library, and

iii) the "Articles" tab on each product page throughout the site.

Here is a link to the video:

http://www.youtube.com/watch?v=tWlpIpj-w6k&list=UUU_RtUa iUgH2DXmieOMTcfg&feature=share&index=6

B. YouTube Channel

Our whole YouTube channel began with short video tutorials demonstrating a particular feature of a chair. Our database has blossomed to over 200 videos at the time of this writing. I have created playlists for each chair model, each playlist containing a series of videos and each video highlighting a different feature.

The scope of our video topics was then broadened to include other topics, including i) interviews with massage chair industry leaders, ii) video journals of visits to massage chair company headquarters and warehouses, iii) massage chair video dictionary terms, iv) video

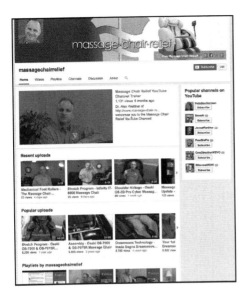

tutorials of certain functions of the website, v) massage chair assembly videos, vi) television appearances and commercials, and, of course, vii) our very popular biweekly *Massage Chair Industry Update*.

You can subscribe to our YouTube channel, *massagechairrelief*, and be the first to be notified of any new videos that are posted on the channel. We typically add one to three new videos each week. The video library keeps growing and providing more and more information… all designed to assist you with your due diligence and, ultimately, choosing the right massage chair.

Here is the link to our YouTube channel:

http://www.youtube.com/user/massagechairrelief

Subscribe today to keep informed!

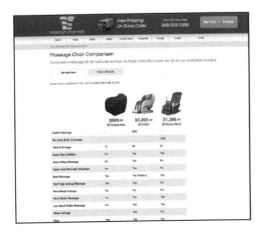

Most Comprehensive Massage Chair Comparison Chart

I began the process of putting together our comparison chart in 2011. It took me three to four months of steady work to complete the project. It has become one of the most frequently visited sections of our website and is used by hundreds of customers each week who are trying to find the right massage chair for them. The data and format have actually been copied and used on other retailer's websites.

You can select any chairs from our database of over 40 massage chair models and compare them feature for feature. The comparison chart is very easy to use and quite intuitive. At the time of this writing, we have close to 60 features we compare for every model we carry. It is a wonderful resource and, again, another must-have for deciding on a massage chair…especially if you cannot actually sit in one in person.

Here is the link to the comparison chart:

http://www.massage-chair-relief.com/massage-chair-comparison/

Free Shipping for All Domestic Massage Chairs

We offer free curbside delivery for every single model we carry to customers within the continental United States. For customers living in Hawaii, Alaska, or anywhere else outside of the continental USA, we can still ship to you, but you will more than likely have additional shipping fees to deal with. We can give you a shipping credit for what we would have spent for free shipping had you lived in the continental USA, which will knock your shipping price down.

We also ship internationally. We have had chair sales to countries all over the world, and we have found that ocean freight offers the most affordable mode of transportation…sometimes surprisingly so. If you are an international customer, we will get you an ocean freight quote (and air freight, if desired, though it's more expensive) and still take care of the shipping logistics from our end.

Rave Customer Reviews

Over the years, we have accumulated quite a plethora of reviews for both our business and our chairs. If you go to the appendix of this book, you will see a section dedicated to customer reviews. But for even hundreds more, go to any product page of any massage chair we carry and check out the "Reviews" section. You will find reviews specific to each particular chair. Many of the reviews also mention the customer's experience with Massage Chair Relief.

We don't mean to brag by telling you about these awesome reviews, but I truly feel that they will help you in your decision-making process. You will love hearing what others have to say about the chair you are possibly interested in as well as what they think about us. I can assure you that each testimonial and review is original and offered without coercion! They will be very helpful in your journey.

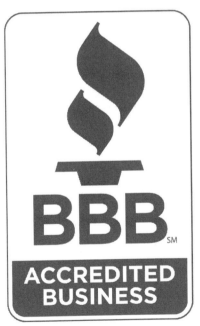

A+ Better Business Bureau Rating

We have been with the BBB since we started and have earned an A+ (top marks) through the years. I take great pride in that because a high ranking indicates a company with integrity and one that takes care of its customers. I feel we do just that. Our attention to customer service is well known in this industry, and that is reflected in our BBB status.

6–18-Month Financing Available

Of course, we accept all major credit cards and bank checks, but we also offer a couple of different options for financing.

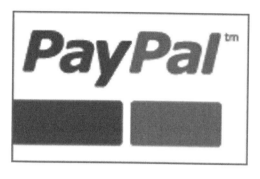

i) PayPal Bill Me Later

The Bill Me Later program from PayPal has become a very popular avenue for customer financing. It is something that can be done from the checkout page on our website. It is very easy to do: you simply log in to your PayPal account from our checkout page and then select the "Bill Me Later" option. PayPal will take care of the rest. When approved, you are eligible for six months of financing with zero percent interest and zero payments.

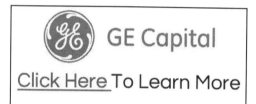

ii) GE Capital

GE Capital offers six- and twelve-month interest-free financing options, but unlike PayPal, they require a minimum monthly payment. You have to download the application form from our website, fill it out, and then submit it to us either by e-mail or fax. We then submit your application to GE, and once approved, we process your order through GE's website. You will then receive your GE Capital card with supporting documentation in the mail.

A few times a year, GE Capital will offer 18 months zero interest financing at a lower processing rate for retailers. That makes it affordable for us to offer that plan to the customer. For example, GE Capital might offer it for one week over the Thanksgiving weekend or for the week of President's Day.

Dr. Weidner's Clinical Chiropractic Experience

Of course, you always have me at your disposal as a resource for your decision-making process. I have years of clinical experience under my belt. I get asked all the time about the ability of a particular model to handle such-and-such a condition or whether any airbags or the rollers will hit this muscle or that ligament. My years of clinical experience qualify me to speak on the physiological effects of massage, particularly as they pertain to massage chairs. You can always tap into my experience and expertise. You can reach me through our toll-free number, 888-259-5380.

Well, there you go! Plenty of reasons to use Massage Chair Relief as your one-stop shop for massage chairs. We try our very best to make it very hard for you to go anywhere else!

In Conclusion...

Well, there you have it—*The Ultimate Massage Chair Buyer's Guide*! I hope you found the information helpful and the decision-making process much, much easier.

If you find that something is not covered in this book at all or to your satisfaction, please feel free to contact me via e-mail at alan@massage-chair-relief.com or by phone, toll-free, at 888-259-5380.

Make sure you check out the appendix beginning on the next page, which is full of very helpful information, including a) helpful and informative massage chair articles, b) a massage chair glossary, c) reviews and testimonials, d) a list of massage therapy contraindications, and e) massage chair resources.

I also invite you to participate on our blog, Facebook page, Google+, and our YouTube channel. Share your experiences, comments, and feedback in those forums for the benefit of other folks who, just like you, are trying to wade through the mountain of information and propaganda that is out there en route to making a very big decision about a very wonderful home therapy.

APPENDIX

a) Article Collection

These are selected articles from our article library. They cover topics that apply to most massage chairs and will assist you in getting a better understanding of what massage chairs are all about. Our article library actually contains hundreds of articles; these are just a few. You can also find articles comparing chair models, reviews of new models, e-mail responses to customers, and news and notes from the massage chair industry.

The following articles were chosen because of their broader appeal to the massage chair shopping audience. You can go to the actual article library to find more articles for your research…

http://www.massage-chair-relief.com/blog/

Shoulder Airbags: What and How

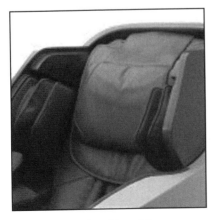

Iyashi shoulder airbags

I think that the first time I ever saw shoulder airbags was on the Panasonic Ep30007 chair. I remember being curious as to why the airbags were in the chair back and pushed the shoulders forward, as this seemed rather counterintuitive to a chiropractor who had worked on correcting forward slumping shoulders. Why on earth would a chair push the shoulders forward when they obviously needed to be pulled back? That was exactly my sentiment when I saw that feature on that chair.

Then, a few years later, Inada introduced the Doctor's Choice 3A massage chair, which had a shoulder housing on either side of the body that had airbags that inflated to the *front* of the shoulders, thereby pinning the shoulders back. Now, that made sense to me. I remember being so impressed with the idea of airbags pinning the shoulders back in an effort to improve posture. I also remember sitting on that chair for the first time and feeling taller (and less slumped when I stood up afterwards. I was excited to have a chair to offer customers that had a feature like this. I felt it was very much needed and that it complemented the spinal correction I did as a chiropractor.

Since that time, we've seen quite a few new models come out with shoulder airbags, but they've not all been the same. A new breed of shoulder airbags came out that only inflated onto the outside aspect of each shoulder (against the deltoid muscles). Their purpose was not to reverse a slumping posture by pinning the shoulders back; they were designed to hold the upper body in place, much like thigh airbags that hold the hips in place, so that the roller massage that passes through the midback region would be accentuated and made more intense by holding the shoulders and upper body immobile. These airbags prevented the rollers from pushing the body forward, thus maximizing the intensity of the roller massage.

Then along came the Inada Sogno that introduced airbags that pushed down from the bottom of the headpiece (aka cervical traction device) onto trapezia muscles at the top of the shoulders. This was a whole different shoulder massage approach. It actually did massage some muscles, whereas the previous shoulder airbag iterations simply compressed against the shoulder joint to hold the body in a particular position.

Here are the three types of shoulder airbags:

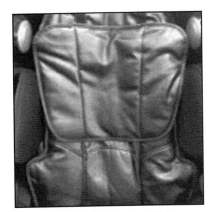

Shoulder Airbags – Side

1. Lateral Compression (side)

These are found in chairs such as the Osaki OS-3D Pro Dreamer, Osaki OS-4000, Panasonic MA70, and Omega Montage Pro. These chairs offer airbags that compress the outer aspect of the shoulders (deltoid muscles) and are designed to hold the upper body in place while the rollers move up and down the spine.

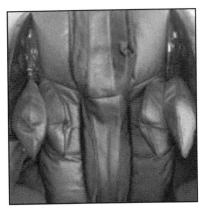

Shoulder Airbags – Front

2. Anterior Compression (front)

These airbags are found in chairs such as the Inada Doctor's Choice (has since been discontinued), Infinity IT-8500, Infinity Iyashi, Osaki OS-3D Pro Cyber, and the Osaki OS-7075R. The purpose of these airbags is twofold: a) to pin the shoulders back for posture correction while the rollers move up and down the spine, and b) to hold the shoulders back during the stretch program. You see, when you are going through the stretch program in a massage chair, the airbags of the foot massager inflate to hold the feet in place while the ottoman drops. Simultaneously, the chair back reclines, thus accentuating the effect of the stretch. With the shoulder airbags inflating to the front of the shoulders, the airbags are doing to the upper body what the foot airbags are doing to the lower body. Both of these airbag features working simultaneously really give the user a great stretch.

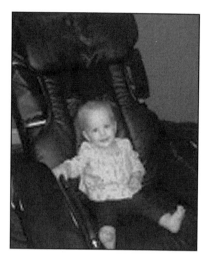

Panasonic EP30007

3. Posterior Compression (rear)

The only chair that has this feature is the Panasonic EP30007, and the only therapeutic benefit I can see from these airbags is a compression against the infraspinatus muscles of the shoulder blades. I suppose you could go so far as to say that it is a trigger-point-like compression of those muscles. You can see the shoulder airbag mechanisms in the picture just above my granddaughter to the left and right of the top of her head.

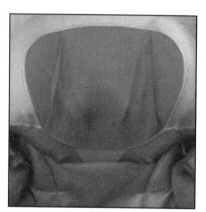

Shoulder Airbags – Top

4. Superior Compression (top)

The Inada Sogno is the only chair that has superior compression, with perhaps the iRobotics 6S chair from Luraco offering something similar. The purpose of these airbags is to impose a compression massage against the muscles at the top of the shoulders (the trapezia muscles). These airbags are not designed for holding or restricting movement of the torso, as with the airbags in #1 and #2 above, but for actual compression massage therapy. You can see on the image to the right the inflated airbags at the bottom of each side of the head piece. These airbags massage the trapezia muscles at the top of your shoulders (commonly affected muscles for desk and computer workers).

I hope this helps you understand what shoulder airbags are and how they work depending on their engineered purpose.

Zero Gravity or Not – That Is the Question!!

Zero gravity has become a very popular feature among massage chair models and with massage chair shoppers. I get asked all the time about whether a particular model has zero gravity or not. The funny thing is, most folks think they want it but have no idea what it really is!

Is zero gravity something that you really want in a massage chair? I will define it and then explain to you the pros and cons of zero gravity, especially as it pertains to you, the user, and your therapeutic experience with or without it in your massage chair.

In physics, zero gravity is defined, essentially, as weightlessness. However, zero gravity as it pertains to seating is defined by two conditions:

1. A 30-degree upward tilt of the seat, and

2. A 120-degree articulation between the tilted seat and the chair back.

The essence of zero gravity in seating is that with these angular articulations, your body and spine are not necessarily in a weightless position (because gravity is always at play here on earth!), but your body is positioned such that it's weight is evenly distributed throughout the body.

Here is a great image of the Human Touch HT-7450, the first zero-gravity massage chair, in its zero-gravity position. Notice the upward tilt of the seat and the angle of the chair back relative to the seat.

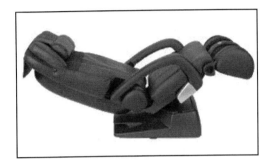

Zero gravity was a feature first introduced by NASA to explain what they found to be the optimal seating position for astronauts who were spending a good amount of their time strapped into their seats in their spaceship as it orbited the earth.

This becomes apparent when you sit in a normal chair with a normal horizontal seat and with a chair back that is either reclined or inclined, and then you put the chair into a zero-gravity position. If you focus on how your low back feels in both positions, you will become very aware of the additional weight, or compression, on the low back when the seat is horizontal. When the zero-gravity positioning is introduced, you will suddenly become aware that the weight or compression on the low back shifts and now feels more evenly distributed throughout the whole body.

That is the benefit of zero gravity in a massage chair. If you have low back pain, either acute or chronic, you will welcome the decompression of the low back that comes with the zero-gravity positioning. This feature is fantastic in a non-massage chair. However, in a massage chair, there is a trade-off, and here it is…

The Reach of the Rollers!

Why is it that a chair like the Inada Sogno, which has only a 29-inch roller track, reaches lower into the buttocks than does a chair like the OS-7075R from Osaki, which has a 31-inch roller track? It's not because the rollers don't go up as high into the neck on the Sogno. The answer is in the seat positioning!

In an April 2013 article, I wrote:

"You see, when the seat remains horizontal, the rollers have a straight shot from the back down to the buttock area. It is a straight line, and the rollers don't have any additional distance to travel other than right from the chair back linearly to the buttock and sacral areas of the seat. On the other hand, the OS-7075R rollers (or the rollers of any massage chair that incorporates zero gravity) need to travel down the distance of the chair back and then, because of the zero-gravity positioning of the seat with its associated 30-degree tilt up, the rollers have to travel around the bend between the chair back and the chair seat and head in a different direction altogether to get to the buttocks area.

"We all know that the shortest distance between two points is a straight line ('as the eagle flies'), and if you add a bend in the line between two points, the distance increases. So when you add a bend in the horizontal line between the chair back and the chair seat, the rollers have a greater distance to travel in the OS-7075R to hit the same areas that the Inada Sogno rollers hit."

And, of course, the rollers in a chair like the OS-7075R do *not* hit the buttocks because they cannot travel that extra distance. I hope this makes sense.

In Summary...

So, going back to the beginning of this article, the trade-off with zero gravity is that if you get the zero-gravity feature, you will have the benefit of relative "weightlessness" or even distribution of body weight, which will take strain and compression off of what might be a very sore low back.

The flip side of the coin is that with zero gravity, the rollers will not reach as far into the buttocks to hit the butt muscles, which is an area that, in most back pain sufferers, could sure use some roller massage. If you get a chair with a horizontal seat, the rollers will do more good lower down into the buttocks region.

You have to decide what is more important to you: decompressing the low back with zero gravity or getting roller massage down into the buttocks. Now, what if there came along a massage chair that had a really long roller track that could overcome the distance hurdle of zero gravity and fully offer roller massage to the buttocks area? Well...it's here. The Infinity Iyashi not only has zero gravity but has a 49-inch roller track, which will go way down into the buttocks area even when zero gravity is being used. I think we are going to see more and more of this extended roller track into the seat idea. Best of both worlds!

Does Osaki Have Backlit Remote Controls?

I recently had a comment on one of my posts asking if the Osaki chairs had backlit remote control buttons. What that means is if there is a light behind each button or behind the remote face as a whole that would allow the user to see the buttons in the dark. This is a legitimate question because many folks use the chair in a dark or poorly illuminated room and have trouble seeing the buttons if they are not backlit.

So I e-mailed Osaki and asked one of their experts if their chairs had backlit remotes. Below is a list of each chair, whether or not its remote is backlit, any additional comment relayed to me by my Osaki contact, as well as images of each remote control. I hope this helps. Each company has a different type of remote, and not all of them are backlit. Perhaps someday I will present a full article going through each company's remote back lighting.

1. **OS-3D Pro Cyber** – "The Cyber chair has the Lit LCD Screen Display, which is a bit larger than some of the other chairs. Also the ON/OFF button lights up. There is a Blue LED bar running across the bottom of the LCD Screen. The individual buttons do not light up."

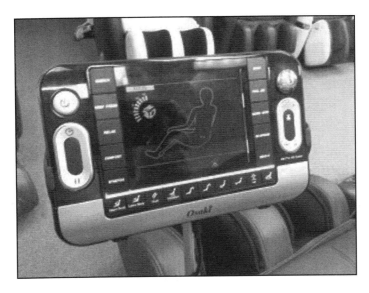

OS-3D Pro Cyber remote

2. **OS-Pro Marquis** – "All buttons light up on the Pro Marquis Chair."

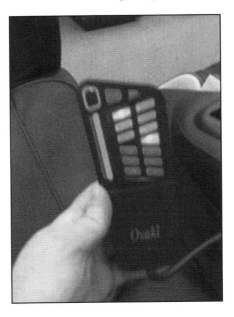

OS-Pro Marquis remote

3. **OS-7075R** – "The OS-7075r control completely lights up."

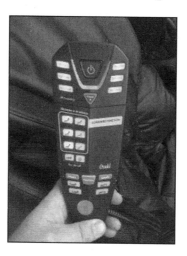

OS-7075R remote

4. **OS-2000 Combo/OS-3000 Chiro** – "LCD Screen lights up and back of remote around buttons in blue. The center buttons are the same for the 3000 Chiro & 2000 Combo. The center button and/or 5th auto program lights up blue, while the other surrounding 4 Auto Programs only light up when you hit the function with a small yellow light."

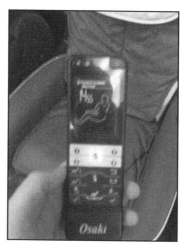

OS-2000 Combo remote

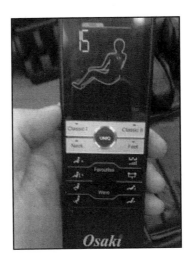

OS-3000 Chiro

5. **OS-4000** – "Only the Auto Programs light up in a sequential order going from top to bottom in that constant order."

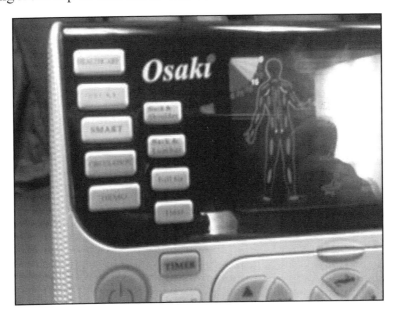

OS-4000 remote

6. **OS-7200H/OS-7200CR/OS-3D Pro Dreamer** – "The LCD screen display of course lights up. The individual buttons with wording light up when you hit the function (i.e., auto programs)."

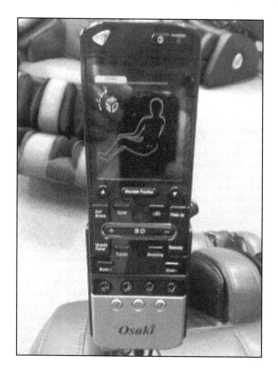

OS-3D Pro Dreamer

Well, there you have it! A good commentary on all the remotes of the Osaki line. Thanks to Chris at Osaki.

Commercial Massage Chair Warranties

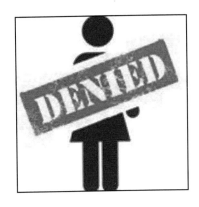

I have been writing an eight-part series of reviews of the warranty coverage of each of the eight companies I represent on my website and store. It is important to note that the discussions in those reviews pertain solely to residential chair placements and use. **What about commercial coverage?** Do the chairs have different coverage if they are placed and used in a business? Well, for the most part, yes they do.

This article will address the commercial coverage offered by each company for their massage chairs. If you use the chair in a business setting where multiple employees and/or customers use the chair, then that would be considered commercial use. If you are buying a chair for your office and you are the principal user of the chair, then the normal warranty would typically apply. Some examples I have seen of commercial use meriting different warranty coverage are spas, salons, tire stores, auto dealerships, employee perks in a business, doctor's offices, dentist's waiting or recovery rooms, retail outlets, gyms, teacher lounges at schools, etc.

I have contacted each of the massage chair companies that I represent, and here are their commercial warranties:

1. Inada

The warranty that comes with one of their chairs is void if used in a commercial setting. You can purchase a commercial warranty for $600 to get the same three-year parts and labor in-home (or should I say in-business?!) coverage for your Inada chair.

If you do not have commercial coverage arranged before purchasing your chair or at least within 30 days of purchasing your chair, your chair warranty will be null and void, and no coverage will be given.

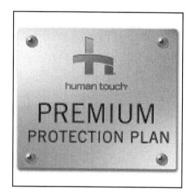

2. Human Touch

Commercial use of the Human Touch chairs will cut your warranty down to 90 days parts and labor in-business and one year parts instead of the usual one year parts and labor in-home and a second year parts that comes with a residential-use chair.

3. Cozzia

Cozzia has no commercial coverage at all. In other words, if you purchase a Cozzia chair for a commercial setting, you will have no coverage at all. Cozzia does not sell or provide any commercial warranty.

4. Panasonic

Panasonic has a very simple, easy-to-understand commercial application of their standard warranty. They offer a standard three-year or 1,000-hour warranty for their MA70, EP30005, and EP30007. If one of these chairs is used in a commercial setting, the 1,000-hour threshold will apply. So if the chair hits 1,000 hours of usage within one year, then the warranty expires at that time. If it lasts two years or three years, then that is the coverage.

I think this is the simplest way to apply a commercial warranty...by the number of hours of usage.

5. Omega

Omega's commercial coverage is one-half of the standard warranty for their chairs. So, for example, their Omega Montage Pro has a five-year parts and labor in-home warranty. If it is used in a commercial setting, the warranty would drop down to two and a half years of coverage. For their chairs that have a one-year parts and labor in-home warranty, such as the Montage Elite or Premier, the warranty coverage would drop down to a half year parts and labor in-home for a commercial setting.

6. Infinity

Infinite Therapeutics offers a two-year parts only commercial warranty. No labor is covered at all.

7. Osaki

The coverage for an Osaki chair in a commercial setting is three years of parts only. No labor is covered. Osaki does, however, offer a caveat for their commercial warranty. If the usage is comparable to a residential setting, which they can see through diagnostic software on the remote control of the chair, Osaki may at their discretion provide labor for the first year.

8. Luraco

Luraco offers six months parts and labor in-store coverage along with one year of parts only. Structure and frame are covered for another year beyond that.

Feel free to call me anytime at 888-259-5380 if you need clarification on any of these commercial or residential warranties. I am always at your disposal.

What Makes Each Massage Chair Unique?

Not all massage chairs are created equally! We carry many different models of massage chairs, and each one has its own unique feature that each company has employed to try to differentiate that chair from the competition. I thought I would make a list of each of our top-selling and/or game-changing chairs and briefly list the features that differentiate them from the rest of the pack or, at the very least, make them unique. Now some of these chairs innovated a technology that was very unique at the time but have since been imitated by others on this list. I will mention both in that case.

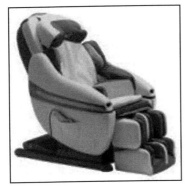
Inada Sogno

1. **Inada Sogno** – I'll start with the granddaddy of massage chairs. The features that still make this chair unique are the airbags in the headpiece that massage the trapezia muscles, innovative body styling (that has been copied ad nauseam by other manufacturers), full arm massage, Dreamwave technology in the seat, 3D massage technology, airbags that massage the iliotibial bands (ITB's), a three-year parts and labor in-home warranty, Japanese-made quality, and a leather upholstery option.

2. **Inada Yume** – Rocking motion of the chair, thera-elliptical kneading in the calves, Japanese-made quality, and lights on the exterior of the chair body (chromotherapy).

3. **Panasonic MA70** – Heated jade rollers, gripping motion of the rollers on top of the shoulders, rotating ottoman and back pad to create a nonmassage chair look, and ITB airbag massage.

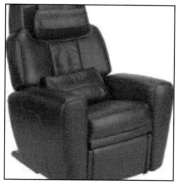

HT-9500

4. **HT-7450** – Zero gravity integrated into the massage chair, obscured calf massage wells, and roller intensity adjustment.

5. **HT-9500x** – Looks like a normal recliner, ottoman that hides underneath the chair seat, roller intensity adjustment, and leather upholstery.

6. **All Human Touch massage chairs** that employ foot and calf massage – Rubber paddles rather than airbags.

7. **Infinity IT-8500** – Mechanical foot rollers, swiveling seat, shoulder airbags that pin the shoulders back (first innovated by Inada in their discontinued Doctor's Choice 3A massage chair), inversion (chair reclines to near horizontal—178 degrees), and MP3 music system.

8. **Infinity Iyashi** – 49-inch roller track that extends down to the buttocks and thighs, unique body styling, sequential arm airbag deployment, TV-like remote control, smartphone app that integrates with a built-in music system, and sliding base.

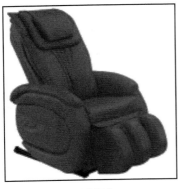

IT-9800

9. **Infinity IT-9800** – True inversion (recline past horizontal—184 degrees), calf swing, no airbags, leather upholstery, and Taiwan-made quality.

10. **Osaki OS-7075R** – Mechanical foot rollers, unique body styling, headband airbag massage, Thai stretch program, and full body heat.

11. **Osaki OS-3D Pro Dreamer** – Mechanical foot rollers, 3D massage technology, domelike cover over back of chair, and music system.

12. **Omega Montage Pro** – Five-year parts and labor in-home warranty, full-body heat, music system, mechanical foot rollers, and foot magnets.

13. **Omega Serenity/Skyline** – Very modern styling without the outward appearance of a massage chair.

14. **iRobotics 6** – Full arm massage, airbags that address the traps, two-year parts and labor in-home warranty, made in the USA, music system, 104 airbags, and 3D massage technology.

Now you have a better idea of what makes each chair unique in comparison to another model. I hope this helps in your massage chair research.

White Glove Delivery - How to Decide if I Need It!

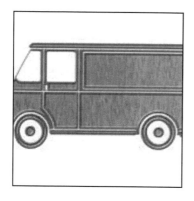

I have touched on this subject before in previous articles, but I want to revisit it here and add some thoughts to the discussion.

There are basically three different shipping options for a massage chair: 1) curbside delivery, 2) threshold delivery, and 3) white glove delivery.

It is probably a good thing to define what *curbside*, *threshold*, and *white glove* mean.

Curbside delivery can quite literally mean dropping off the chair on the easement by your home! Most delivery folks will at least put the chair in your driveway or somewhere on your property closer to your door, but by pure definition, curbside means just that...dropping off the chair right by the curb.

Threshold delivery means that the delivery team will cross the threshold of your home and put the chair inside your doorway.

White glove delivery is a service offered wherein the delivery team not only brings your new massage chair into your home, but they will also bring it to the room in which you want the chair set up, unpack it, assemble it, and then get rid of all the packing material for you. The only thing you have to do is sit in your new chair and turn it on. White glove delivery people *do not* offer tips on how to operate the chair or give you operating instructions. You are on your own once the chair is set up.

All of our chairs come with standard curbside delivery. Panasonic has even recently added threshold delivery to all of their chairs as the standard delivery. White glove delivery has a charge associated with it ($199.99).

The question I get asked most is whether a customer will need the white glove service or not, which translates to "is it really worth it to me to pay that extra $200 for white glove delivery?" Here are some suggestions that I have gleaned from dealing with massage chairs and their associated deliveries for almost ten years:

1. If you are unable to lift 200+ pound boxes and do not have any younger bodies around to do the heavy lifting for you, white glove delivery might be an option for you.

2. If you are completely inept at assembling mechanical things, feel completely and utterly intimidated by mechanical things, feel no confidence whatsoever in putting anything together, and don't have anyone available who does, then you might consider white glove delivery.

3. If you love the challenge of putting something together and you can get the chair box(es) into your home from the outside, then you don't need to spend the extra money to get the white glove delivery.

Here are a few more things to consider when dealing with the massage chair shipping/delivery issue:

a) It is most likely the case that the folks doing the white glove service for you have never assembled the chair before and are as unfamiliar with it as you are.

b) If putting the chair together is not intimidating to you in the least but you have no way of getting the heavy box(es) into your home, I might suggest asking the delivery guys if they would bring it across your threshold to at least get the chair into your home. If that doesn't work, then try offering the drivers $20 or so to bring the chair in for you. You might even get them to bring it to the room in which you want it placed. Most of these folks are quite decent and would be willing to do that for a few extra bucks "under the table."

c) Once the chair boxes are in the designated room of your house, you will still need another person to help lift the chair body out of the box to do the final assembly. It is too heavy to do it alone.

d) Many chairs require very little assembly...maybe nothing more than zipping on a zipper or attaching the armrests. That is stuff that even I can do! And I must be honest—I fall under the category of "pretty useless" when it comes to assembling mechanical things. However, more of the newer chairs come in multiple boxes, most commonly a box for the chair body and a box or two with the arm-rests and ottoman. These are tougher and more time-consuming to put together. I personally don't do real well with assembling these multiple-boxed chairs.

Find out from us when you buy the chair how difficult the assembly is so that you can determine if you think it is easy enough for you. If so, then you will just need some bodies, whether it is the delivery guys whom you offer $20 to, your kids or neighbors, or your spouse, to help lift the chair box(es) into your home. Then you can do the rest.

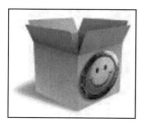

e.) If there is even a remote possibility that you may return your chair, keep all the boxes and packaging material. If you don't sendyour chair back in the original packaging, your return shipping costs will be even more through the roof than they already are! Once you are sure that you are keeping your chair, go ahead and do with the packaging what you will.

I hope this article makes the delivery options clear and helps you decide if the white glove delivery option is right for you.

A Chair for a 4'10" Petite Woman?

I often have calls and inquiries about which chairs would be best suited for tall folks, but once in a while, I get an e-mail like this one asking for chair suggestions for someone quite short.

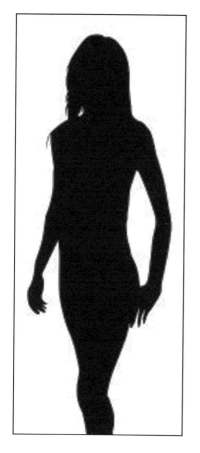

Hi, Dr. Weidner, I found your site while researching for a massage chair for my mom. Your website and reviews are truly great, the best I could find on Google. My mom is very petite, only 4'10" tall. She has lower back pain close to the spine. I really want to get her a massage chair to alleviate her pains. I'm wondering which models would fit her better. I've seen some good reviews about Osaki models; would Osaki 7200h fit her size? I also saw a human touch model in Costco; that chair looks pretty small but doesn't have as many fancy functionalities as Osaki does. Could you please give some suggestions on which brand/model would work better for her case? I'd really appreciate it. Thanks, Liang

My Response:

Hi, Liang.

Thank you so much for your inquiry. There are certainly some chairs that would fit your mom better than others. I will make some recommendations, but first let me discuss the OS-7200 massage chair from Osaki.

The OS-7200 is a chair built to fit larger body frames. It is a wonderful chair, but it was built to cater to the taller and bigger folks who don't fit in the OS-4000 very well. The features of the OS-7200 are fantastic, but it would probably feel too large for your petite mom.

Although there are not many chairs that I carry that are specifically designed to accommodate a 4'1" height, here are some chair models that come pretty close:

1. **Inada Sogno** – This chair states a height reference of 4'11". It also has a Youth program that caters to that lower height. This is a very expensive chair and widely considered the best chair in the world, so it may not fit within your budget. It is also known for a more gentle and soothing massage, which may be just perfect for your mother's petite frame.

2. **Panasonic EP30007** – This chair actually accommodates a frame as short as 4'6". It does not handle anyone over 6' all that well, especially if you have longer legs, but it might be fabulous for your mom. It has an aggressive massage, but it can be adjusted in intensity. It also has arm and leg/foot massage airbags and a voice command that makes it easy to understand how to use.

You could also consider the EP30005, which is a sister model to the EP30007. Panasonic's 1285 also has the same height support as the other two. It just doesn't have the same rich feature set as the 30005 and 30007 models.

3. **Infinity IT-8500 and IT-8200** – Wonderful chairs that can fit someone at 4'11" quite comfortably. They are very popular models and can also cater to tall folks. Mechanical foot rollers make these chairs unique. The massage is more vigorous with these two models, and that intensity cannot be adjusted except with the use of a back pad or folded throw blanket.

4. **Infinity IT-7800** – A basic chair, but it caters to a frame as short as 4'9" tall. Good chair but without the large number of airbags you'll find in the IT-8500 and IT-8200.

5. **ZeroG 4.0** – A great chair from Human Touch that can cater to the shorter frame. This chair, as do all Human Touch chairs, has a fabulous foot and calf massage in the ottoman, which hides underneath the chair seat. The roller intensity can be adjusted in both the low back and neck regions, which will allow your mother some flexibility for comfort.

6. **Osaki OS-3000** – This chair is great for shorter frames as well as taller ones but has a roller track that goes down into the buttocks to really address low back issues well. All of the above-mentioned chairs also do quite well in the low back, but the OS-3000 has a 36-inch roller track, which is a good 5–6 inches longer than the longest of the others.

I hope these suggestions help in some way. Let me know if I can assist you in any other way.

Over 6' Tall and 300 Pounds –
Which Chair Might Work for You?

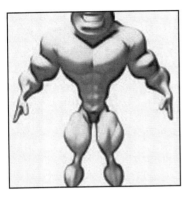

Things just come in waves. In the course of two to three days, I had three inquiries from customers that had to do with size and weight and which chair would work. I had two folks who were over six feet and weighed between 300 and 350 pounds. On one of the days when I received an inquiry, I had a salesman at the showroom who overheard me talking on the phone with this customer about his size concerns. The salesman just happened to be 6'5" tall and weigh 350 pounds, and he just happened to offer to sit in all of my massage chairs in the showroom and give his honest opinion on which chairs fit OK and which did not.

Before I go into the results, I should say that this fellow, named Lyle, was very tall, and his weight was quite evenly distributed. He had a big belly, but the remainder of his frame was evenly distributed. There are different body shapes and sizes, so what might fit for Lyle may not work exactly for someone who has exceedingly broad shoulders or a massive midsection or buttocks. Does that make sense? So Lyle's opinions are for his body type and may or may not work for yours. But at least these are some helpful suggestions and opinions that may serve you in your decision-making process.

Here is a list of the chairs he tried and a concise opinion of each as they pertained to his size and fit:

Osaki OS-7075R – too tight in the shoulders

Osaki OS-7200H – arms and shoulders too tight

Panasonic MA70 – too tight in seat and shoulders

Panasonic 30007 – too tight in seat and too short of a chair

IT-8200 – too tight in shoulders

IT-9800 – fit OK

iRobotics 6 – too tight in shoulders and body

HT-7450 – fit OK

HT-9500x – fit OK

Inada Yume – fit OK

Inada Sogno – fit OK (his exact terms were "Oh, wow" and "Unbelievable")

So the long and short of it is that the following chairs fit him:

IT-9800

HT-7450

HT-9500x

Inada Yume

Inada Sogno

Each chair company has a recommended weight maximum of the user. Infinite Therapeutics IT-9800 has a weight limit of 350 pounds. The weight limit for the HT-7450 and HT-9500x is 285 pounds. The motto for Inada chairs is "if you can fit, you can sit." So, using recommended weights, the IT-9800 and the Inada chairs would be the best options for a person of Lyle's size.

I hope this helps somewhat in deciding which massage chair to get when you have a bigger body type.

5 Tips to Help You Decide Which Chair Is Right for You!

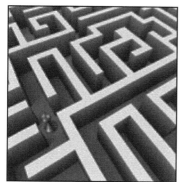

Making the decision of which massage chair to buy is a heavy one— so many chairs to pick from, so many models, so many colors, so many features. Even if you have a chance to sit in a chair, it is still hard to decide, especially if you have other models to try out at the same time.

Very confusing business. I get calls all day long about the differences among massage chairs and massage chair companies. Here are some suggestions when deciding which chair to get or which one may be right for you:

1. **What are your needs?** Do you have low back pain, upper back pain, headaches, neck pain, butt pain, midback pain?...and the list goes on and on. Or are you just getting a chair for stress relief, for the novelty of having one, for a theater room, or for something else besides some pain relief?

2. **What features are a must-have in your opinion?** Do you want foot rollers, which have become all the rage lately for massage chair shoppers? Do you want a music system? Is heat important to you? Do you want lots of airbags? Do you want a chair with adjustable intensity for the rollers and the airbags? How about intensity...do you want something that will rock your world because it is so intense, or do you want a gently soothing massage instead? Do you want a chair that can handle a large body frame? Do you want zero gravity,

head massage, upper arm massage, rocking, foot massage?...and the list goes on and on. Figure out what you want and need, and then it will be easier to siphon through all the models out there to find the one that most closely meets all your wants and needs.

Is it important to you if a chair is made in Japan, China, or the USA?

3. **What is your budget?** If price is a barrier to entry into this market, then there are some models you don't even want to look at. On the other hand, is money not an object to you and you want the best chair out there? Then there are some models you certainly want to include in your research. You can get massage chairs priced anywhere from $1,500 to $8,000!

4. **Compare features!** You can do that easily enough with a good massage chair comparison chart. Compare each model and decide which one sounds like it would fit your needs the very best. Here is a fantastic comparison chart to get you started (I think it's the best dang comparison chart in the industry!):

http://www.massage-chair-relief.com/massage-chair-comparison/

A lot of the models out there are very, very similar in looks and feature sets. It is good to be able to compare each model to see where the subtle differences are.

5. **Try out as many as you can!** Now, this is a hard one. Other than our showroom store, Massage Chair Relief in Salt Lake City, Utah, good luck finding a place where you can have all the major name brands under one roof to try out. But if you can, at the very least, try out one or two models on your list; that will help immensely.

I am of the opinion, based on ten years of personal experience in this industry, that no matter how much studying you do on paper or on the Internet to compare features, there is nothing quite like actual in-chair experience to figure out which chair is right for you. I can't tell you how many folks have come to my showroom from all over the country believing that they knew which chair they wanted but just needed to sit in it to confirm their decision...and found out that the chair they thought they wanted, based on their online research, was not at all what they were expecting. And they decided on another model in our showroom.

We have actually begun a program for out-of-staters that encourages folks from all over the country to come to our showroom to try out all of our 14 display models. And lots of folks are taking us up on the offer. Here is more info on that program:

http://www.massage-chair-relief.com/out-of-state.html

You can see that there are lots of things to consider when deciding on a massage chair. I hope this assists you in some way in your decision-making process.

Study: Which Massage Chair Is the Loudest?

I had an interesting e-mail a few weeks back from a fellow who wanted to buy a new massage chair but was concerned about how loud it would be in his bedroom. He wanted to use it after his wife went to bed and didn't want a loud chair that would awaken her from her slumber.

I went down to the showroom to listen to the chair he was interested in, and it seemed quiet enough. But I had no objective way to tell him how loud or quiet the chair actually was.

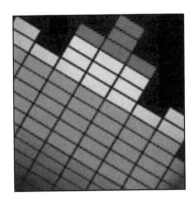

A customer of mine, Phill Ruhnke, was visiting our showroom from the Chicago area, and I mentioned this customer's request to him. He suggested downloading an app onto my cell phone that would measure the decibels (db) of a massage chair—in other words, quantitatively measure how loud a massage chair truly is. I thought it was a fantastic idea!

I immediately downloaded an app called Sound Meter and became familiar with it in quite short order. Over the last two days, I have been measuring the db levels of almost every massage chair in our showroom. I am going to present my findings to you in this blog post.

The ground rules for this little research project...

1. I measured the db level while sitting in each massage chair holding the cell phone and downloaded app approximately six inches from my face.

2. I began measuring the db levels after the scan on each chair was completed and an auto program had begun.

3. I chose one auto program per chair and tried to select the one program that seemed to be the most aggressive and that used air-bags more rapidly. I hypothesized that the most aggressive program would also be the loudest.

4. I measured the db levels for a period of anywhere from three to five minutes and annotated the lowest and highest db's found during that time frame.

5. Ambient noise was not eliminated, but I did all in my power to minimize it; i.e., the air conditioning/heating unit was turned off; my cell phone was put on mute; and I did the measurements during the day when traffic outside of our showroom was at its lowest point during the day (not during morning and afternoon traffic).

6. All neck, head, and low back pillows were removed so that my head was immediately adjacent to the rollers. I did not remove head-pieces that had airbags built into the pillows, i.e., Inada Sogno, Osaki OS-7200H, and IT-8200.

Here are the results of the testing (I will list the model of the chair, the program chosen, and the db range as displayed by the Sound Meter app):

1. Inada Sogno – "Morning" Program – *44–68 db*

2. Inada Yume – "Rock & Massage" Program – *51–63 db*

3. Osaki OS-7075R – "Weightless" Program – *50–73 db*

4. Human Touch HT-9500 – Program #1 – *56–61 db*

5. Human Touch HT-7450 – Program #1 – *53–63 db*

6. Human Touch ZeroG 4.0 – "Refresh" Program – *54–64 db*

7. Luraco iRobotics 6 – "Japanese" Program – *53–72 db*

8. Osaki OS-7200H – "Wake Up" Program – *43–71 db*

9. Panasonic MA70 – "Deep" Program – *36–68 db*

10. Panasonic EP30007 – "Deep" Program – *41–65 db*

11. Infinity IT-8200 – "Refresh" Program – *48–68 db*

In order to give a decent frame of reference of what these db numbers mean, I will mention that at complete relative silence (some very minor ambient noise), the reading of the app was 32 db. The db range in a room with normal human talking was between 82–90 db.

Here are some things gleaned from this data:

1. Every chair made some level of audible noise, with the Panasonic MA70 registering the lowest db level during its program.

2. The chairs that had fewer airbags—i.e., Inada Yume, HT-9500, and HT-7450—registered the lowest numbers at the high end of the db ranges.

3. Conversely, the massage chairs that had the most airbags—i.e., Inada Sogno, Osaki OS-7075R, Osaki OS-7200H, and iRobotics 6—registered the highest numbers at the high end of the db ranges.

4. The two Panasonic models had the lowest numbers at the low end of the db ranges.

5. The three Human Touch models, along with the iRobotics 6, had the highest numbers at the low end of the db ranges.

6. The smallest ranges between high and low belonged to the three Human Touch chairs.

7. The widest range between high and low belonged to the Panasonic MA70.

I found that three things contributed to "noise" as interpreted by the Sound Meter app: a) the motors, b) airbag deployment, and c) the sound of the rollers rubbing against the chair's upholstery.

False Positives

Every study has variables that are hard to completely control and might skew the numbers somewhat. In this little study, a couple of those factors would be:

a) Not a fixed distance between my face and the phone position (I did not measure each placement exactly, and my hand did tend to move with fatigue the longer the testing period went).

b) Ambient noise from the street or from attached neighboring retail space. This app is quite sensitive, and I don't know how much outside noise it actually picked up, even though I may not have noticed any changes with my own ears while I was focused on the readings.

c) I did not test every program on each chair, nor did I test one program all the way through its preprogrammed timer.

Conclusion

Before I began this little research study, my experience with these chairs led me to believe that the iRobotics 6 would be the noisiest chair. My assumption was close, as the Osaki OS-7075R was the highest at 73 db, with the iRobotics 6 coming in at a close second with 72 db.

Despite these ranges, I must say that all of these chairs are relatively quiet. I don't think that many of them would awaken a sound sleeper at all. Some might disturb a light sleeper at some point during the program.

Massage Chair Roller Track Length and the Low Back

The length of the roller track in a massage chair determines how high and how low the rollers will travel along your spine. It goes without saying that the longer the roller track, the more of

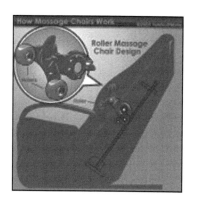

http://electronics.

howstuffworks.com/

gadgets/home/

massage-chair1.htm

your spine will get massaged by the rollers. For example, the Panasonic MA70 has a roller track of 31 inches, whereas the HT-7450 from Human Touch has a roller track length of only 24 inches. When you sit on the two chairs one after the other and compare the feel of the rollers, it is obvious that the rollers of the HT-7450 do a great job reaching the top of the neck but get down only to the belt line of the low back area.

The Panasonic MA70 with its 31-inch track, on the other hand, also reaches up to the base of the skull at the top end of the roller track, but it hits the buttocks and sacral area very well. When comparing these two chair models, one can see that the difference in length of the roller track is felt primarily in the low back area. The HT-7450 goes only as low as the belt line; the Panasonic MA70 gets down into the buttocks.

Now, let me muddy the waters a bit. When you sit on the Panasonic MA70 and then compare its roller's reach to that of the Osaki OS-7075R, which also has a 31-inch roller track, why does it feel like the rollers hit the buttocks on the MA70 but it doesn't feel like they go that low on the OS-7075R? This is something you notice when you test both of them side by side.

Zero gravity is the answer to that question!

Part of the zero-gravity feature in a massage chair is that the seat of the chair tilts up 30 degrees from horizontal. The OS-7075R has the zero-gravity feature; therefore, its seat tilts up. The Panasonic MA70 does not have the seat tilting feature, so its seat remains horizontal. You may be asking, "What does this have to do with anything?" Well, a lot when it comes to getting a massage deeper down into the buttocks area.

You see, when the seat remains horizontal, the rollers have a straight shot from the back down to the buttocks area. It is a straight line, and the rollers don't have any additional distance to travel other than right from the chair back linearly to the buttock and sacral areas of the seat. On the other hand, the OS-7075R rollers need to travel down the distance of the chair back, and then, because of the zero-gravity positioning of the seat with its associated 30-degree tilt up, the rollers have to travel around the bend between the chair back and the chair seat and head in a different direction altogether to get to the buttocks area.

We all know that the shortest distance between two points is a straight line ("as the eagle flies"), and if you add a bend in the line between two points, the distance increases. So when you add a bend in the horizontal line between the chair back and the chair seat (i.e., a 30-degree bend!), the rollers have a greater distance to travel in the OS-7075R to hit the same areas that the Panasonic MA70 rollers hit. But since both chairs have only the same 31-inch roller tracks to work with, the MA70 track reaches further down into the buttocks because the rollers don't have as far to travel. The rollers of the OS-7075R have to travel around the bend, which keeps the 31-inch track from reaching as low as the straight shot of the MA70.

Does that make sense? I hope I have explained it satisfactorily.

The long and short of this message is...if you want the rollers of your new massage chair to reach further down into your buttocks and sacral area, then you'd better consider two things:

1. Make sure the track is as long as it can be (and 31 inches is the longest track we have seen so far), and

2. Decide if zero gravity is more important than getting your buttocks massaged, because you can't have both...at least not with the massage chair technology we have at our disposal today.

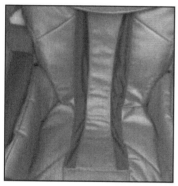

Iyashi roller track

UPDATE: As of 08/26/13, Infinite Therapeutics has come out with a new model, the Iyashi, which boasts a 49-inch roller track!! It is the longest I've seen...by far. The massage in the buttocks and pelvis is unparalleled. I just love it.

Top of Shoulder Massage - Which Chairs Have It?

When people ask me about whether a chair gives a good shoulder massage, I always have to ask, "What do you mean by 'shoulder'?" You see, a shoulder to one person could mean between the shoulder blades, to another it could mean the outside of the shoulders (where the deltoid muscles are), and yet to another person the shoulder could mean the shoulder blades themselves.

For today's article, I am going to chat about the top of the shoulder, or the location of the trapezia muscles. There are not many chairs that cater to this part of the spine, but those that do, do a nice job.

I just love having my trapezia muscles massaged by a licensed massage therapist. If you work at a computer all day, you know what I am talking about. Those dang muscles get so tight that a massage is exactly what you need at the end of a long day. Those tight muscles are often part of the whole stress headache syndrome. It is painful to have them massaged, but man, do they feel great after a massage, along with everything else from the neck up.

There are two ways that a massage chair can address this area...one is with the rollers, and the other is with the airbags. Let's talk about rollers first.

Roller Massage

All massage chairs nowadays have an S-shaped roller track that rolls along the contours of the spine. That is to say, the rollers go more forward into the lumbar or low back spine and the cervical spine or neck, and those same rollers retract a bit for the midback or thoracic spine. When those rollers go up from the midback to the upper back and then on to the neck, the rollers pretty much stay on track with the spine and miss the trapezia muscles altogether.

Panasonic, however, has come up with a pretty interesting twist to the roller system to address a portion of the trap muscles. When those rollers come up the upper back between the shoulder blades and start moving up to the neck, rather than going straight onto the neck, the rollers pause a bit, roll forward onto the levator scapulae (the muscles at the top of the shoulder blades), and then on to the posterior portion of the traps. Those rollers stay for a few moments on those particular muscles and work out the knots.

And do they ever work on those knots! Depending on how tight your muscles are, you will squirm a bit when those rollers hit those muscle knots. In the biz, we call those knots *trigger points*, and massage is the way to release them. The Panasonic MA70 does this masterfully. I love how those heated jade rollers hit those muscles and work them into submission. Once the rollers have done their thing, they move on up to the neck and skull.

Panasonic calls this motion *grasping*, and it feels as if those rollers are grabbing a hold of those muscles and shaking out the knots. I love it, and I'm sure you would love it, too. Panasonic is the only company I know that has rollers that actually do this particular motion.

Airbag Massage

The Inada Sogno Dreamwave massage chair pioneered the airbag massage feature back in 2008, and the only other chair that I am aware of that uses airbags to massage the trapezia muscles is the Osaki OS-7200H. Here is what they do…

If you look at both chairs, you'll see that they each have a headpiece. Built into the headpiece is an airbag system that inflates down onto the top of the shoulders where the trapezia muscles are located. The airbags on the Sogno hit the spot with more finesse and specificity, but both chairs offer that feature. You can adjust the intensity of the airbag compression to cater to different sensitivities. The compression of the airbags onto the traps causes the muscles to reflexively relax after the compression is over. It is a very clever way to approach this area of the body.

The airbags hit a greater portion of the traps, whereas the rollers of the Panasonic MA70 hit more of the posterior portion of the muscles (the back part, that is!). Both feel quite different, and trying them both out is the best way to know which one will work best for your body and your threshold of discomfort.

Customer Warranty Support – What Should You Expect?

One of the things that I hold most dear in my relationship with my customers is the ability to tell them that the chair they are buying is backed by a massage chair company with a great warranty. It is so important to me that my customers have the best support available when they buy a chair from me because they are committing thousands of dollars, often sight unseen, to a chair that is supposed to bring them pain and stress relief.

Nothing brings me as a retailer greater joy than to hear that my customer who is having an issue with a chair is getting well taken care of by the company that makes or imports the chair and that the problem is being or has been resolved. It should not be a surprise to anyone that sometimes things go wrong with an electronic/mechanical device. It happens to new cars all the time...it also happens, once in a while, to massage chairs. But it is the response of the massage chair company to my customer's problem that makes or breaks the experience, in my honest opinion.

Nothing brings me more misery and consternation as a retailer than hearing that my customer is frustrated because a problem with his or her chair is not getting fixed. I always counsel my customers to call me and get me involved in the process if they are having a problem with their chair *and* having a problem getting good tech support from the company that made or imported their chair. I want my customers taken care of...abundantly well! I will get a call once in a while from a frustrated customer—sometimes friendly, sometimes quite ticked off—who says that he or she contacted such-and-such massage chair company to get a problem fixed or a part replaced and then weeks later still had heard nothing from the company. I can't tell you how irritated I get when I get a call or e-mail from a customer telling me that!

I will get involved and write e-mails or make phone calls to make sure my customer is being taken care of. It seems to help quite a bit when I do get involved. What bugs me, though, is that I should never really have to get involved. If the massage chair company is doing its job in the face of a problem with *their* chair, I should never hear anything except "they took care of it, Dr. W." But that is not always the case.

Obviously, sometimes it is a misunderstanding or a timing issue, but what chaps my hide is when complaints are forgotten or ignored (perhaps hoping the customer will go away?) or when a company is unwilling to take responsibility for an issue that is clearly theirs.

Most of the massage chair companies for whom I sell have a tech/warranty support department that will handle your call immediately or, at the very least, the same day. A couple of the companies do not have a department per se but have sales reps or company principals who will handle the support calls. It doesn't matter to me how they have their infrastructure set up as long as they take care of my customers as seamlessly as possible.

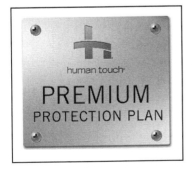

I must say that I have been very impressed with the support given to my customers by Human Touch, Inada, and Infinite Therapeutics. Panasonic has good support, but sometimes it is hard to get set up with a local authorized service center, as I have discussed in previous posts. I have not had any experience with Cozzia yet, so I will reserve judgment on that company. It is sometimes hard to get a hold of Omega, but they have taken care of my customers as far as

I am aware when communication is established. You usually have to leave a message with them, and they will get back to you within a day or two. Osaki takes care of my customers, but sometimes it takes a long, long time and a lot of follow-up by yours truly and by my customer. That can be very frustrating.

Remember, if you are my customer and you find that you are having difficulty getting assistance from the company that manufactured or imported your chair, let me know and I'll get involved with calls and e-mails. I will make sure you are taken care of.

Oh, and before I forget, if you are happy or unhappy with the support you received from a massage chair company, please feel free to leave a review of your experience with the chair and the company. Just go to the product page of your chair on our site and scroll down the page to find the Reviews section and share your experience with the rest of the world. Your review will be very helpful for other massage chair shoppers.

How to Keep Your New Chair Healthy and Happy!

So you've got your new massage chair, and you want to take good care of it. What should you be doing on a regular basis to keep it functioning at its best? Well, not much, believe it or not. Here are some tips to keeping your chair functioning optimally and looking good for years to come:

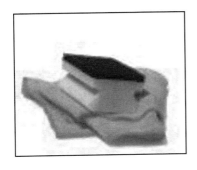

1. Unlike a car, you do not have to perform regular service—i.e., tune-ups, lube jobs, etc.—on your new massage chair. The mechanical side of the chair is all self-sustaining. Everything it needs to run for years is already included in the chassis of the chair. Do not even attempt to get inside of the chair and put grease or any type of lubrication on the gears or motors. Just don't touch it. Should you require a new part in the guts of the chair and if for some reason that new part needs lubrication, let the technician do it or follow the tech support advice to do so.

2. **Cleaning the upholstery** is probably the biggest maintenance thing you could do for your chair. What is recommended is using a luke-warm water solution with some mild detergent and a soft cloth to wipe down the exterior of your chair. No doubt you will get some scuffs and smudges on your chair, but cleaning it is not a big deal... it's very easy to do on all leather and synthetic leather upholsteries.

The tech guy at Inada, Brandon, says they spray Windex on a soft cloth and wipe down the chairs with that. I would never have guessed Windex, but that's what works for them. He also recommends staying away from alcohol-based cleaners or other household cleaners because of the toxic chemicals and abrasives typically found in these types of cleaners. These types of cleaners can cause scratching on the finish or cracking of the material. It might also cause the color to fade on the material.

If you have a cleaner that you're interested in using—e.g., some vinyl cleaner—and aren't sure of what it will do to your chair's upholstery, try using it on a small section that is not readily visible and see if it has an adverse affect on the material.

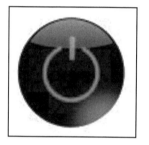

3. For a number of years, we used a simple leather cleaner/conditioner on our leather-upholstered chairs. I did not see any ill effects of using that type of a cleaner on that premium material.

4. Use a **surge protector**! I have seen firsthand what an electrical storm and power outage can do to a massage chair. We've seen a few blowouts over the years and have learned to spend a few bucks to get a surge protector. I think we got one at a local store for only $10 or so—a little investment that pays off huge in an electrical storm.

5. If you have kids or grandkids who tend to be rather destructive with electronic gadgets, as many of mine are, I would suggest unplugging the power cord or locking up the chair with the included key (if yours comes with one) so that your delightful offspring don't get on the chair and summarily destroy it. Kids have a knack for doing things to electronic devices that were never dreamed of by the

inventors of that product. If there is a previously unheard-of way to destroy a product…a child will find it!

Well, that's about it for maintaining a healthy and happy chair. If you have any additional suggestions, please feel free to add them in the comment section of this blog post.

Problem with a New Massage Chair? Rule #1 - Don't Freak Out!

When I was a younger man, just after getting married, I took a job at a car dealership. The dealership sold new Hondas. The Honda was one of the most reliable cars on the road, yet once in a while, there was a problem with a brand-new car that required the new owner to bring the car down to the dealership so that the service department could do the repair...all under warranty, of course.

This proved to be something of an inconvenience for the customer because it took time from the customer's life to come down to the dealership and leave the car there for a day or two. However, I don't remember a lot of grumbling about it. It is just what you do...if there is a problem with a new car, you bring it in and get it fixed under warranty. Easy peasy, lemon squeezy. Standard operating procedure.

Well, this may blow your mind, but occasionally a new massage chair may have a problem with it that requires a new part or, heaven forbid, a complete chair replacement. Almost all of the massage chairs that we carry on our site have, at the very least, a one-year parts and labor in-home warranty. So should something go wrong with your new chair, the company responsible for the chair will send you a part and a technician to repair the problem or replace the part. Sometimes you may be put out by having to send back the damaged part once the chair is fixed so that the company can figure out why the part didn't work and then make it right for the next shipment from China or Japan.

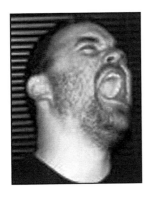

This doesn't sound too problematic, especially when you compare it to having to bring a car in and leaving it for a day or two while also needing to arrange a ride home or to work from the dealership.

It amazes me how wound up some folks get when a chair has what is usually just a small issue that needs remedying when the chair is unpacked and assembled. It is rare, but once in a while, it happens. Sometimes it may even take a couple of tries to get the chair working, particularly if the technician and the company can't figure out the problem right away. *That* is what the warranty is for...just like the car. This does not mean you have a lemon!!!

Now, just because you get a new Honda that has a slight problem, that doesn't mean the car you have is a piece of junk. After the repair, it may be just perfect...like new...as if nothing was ever wrong with it. Your massage chair is no different. Quality components are covered under warranty. If the chair ends up being a total and complete lemon, guess what? The company will replace the chair for you. I wouldn't carry the companies I do if I didn't think they'd take care of you no matter what happens to your chair.

Cars and chairs are made up of electronic components with lots and lots of circuitry. It is quite possible that something could be amiss when you get your chair. But don't worry...the warranty that comes with the new equipment will cover it. I figure it is much better to have something go wrong with your new chair while it is under warranty than two years later when most warranties have expired.

So once in a great while, I have a customer who insists that the chair is no good because a small part is not working when he or she sets up the chair...*and he or she hasn't even given the massage chair company a chance to fix it!!!!!* The customer wants to return the chair. Now the client has to ship the chair back to us and pay for shipping as well as pay for credit card fees from the original transaction when the refund is issued. I may be a simpleton, but man, that seems like such an expensive overreaction to something that could be remedied with a simple part replacement…at no monetary cost to the customer.

Oh well…I'm glad I got that off my chest, and I hope it puts your mind at rest when ordering a new chair. Not every single chair is 100% perfect 100% of the time. Sometimes it may require a little additional attention. But you know what? The massage chair company will make it right. They will fix it. They want their chairs and their company to have a good reputation. It is in their best interest to make sure you are happy. It is also in *my* best interest to make sure you are happy, so I will assist in any way I can to make sure you are taken care of.

Just sayin'…

10 Cool Massage Chair Features (Part 1)

I was just thinking about some of the cool and unique functions and features that I see on some of the chairs I carry. It is amazing to me how interesting and innovative some of these features are. Pretty smart designers and engineers have made the massage chair industry a lot of fun. I will discuss ten things between Part 1 and Part 2 of this article.

Here are the first five things I've found to be kinda cool in some of the chairs we carry:

1. Headband Airbag Massage

I'd never seen the headband airbag massage feature before, and, to be quite honest, I didn't think too much about it when I first saw it in the Osaki OS-7075R. It looked a little cumbersome and almost looked like it didn't belong. But after trying it out, I thought it was quite the cool feature. It uses airbags to squeeze the temporal muscles and the suboccipitals (under the back of the skull). For headache sufferers, this is a useful tool. And the squeeze is not light…it is quite vigorous. The headband has two hard rubber nodules in the back to work those suboccipital muscles. When the airbags compress those nodules, the headband had better be situated correctly or else you get those two hard rubber nodules digging into your skull! When this thing is worn right, it can certainly do some stress headache sufferers some good.

2. **Foot Rollers**

Foot rollers are becoming increasingly popular in newer massage chair models. It makes sense especially for plantar fasciitis sufferers. It can feel a little intense at first, but once you get used to it, you will adore it. Foot rollers combined with airbag or paddle foot massage can be quite therapeutic, with or without a musculoskeletal issue. Chairs that boast mechanical foot rollers in one form or another include the IT-8100, IT-8200, IT-8500, Omega Montage Pro, Osaki OS-7075R, and ZeroG 4.0.

3. **Dreamwave Technology**

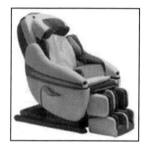

Inada Sogno

Inada introduced Dreamwave technology with the Sogno in 2008. It was the first time we'd seen a chair seat do more than just inflate. With this feature, the chair seat moves from side to side and up and down. For a hot low back problem, I can't think of a better way to address it than a passive seat motion. Folks who use the chair love the Dreamwave feature because it tends to be quite relaxing. The IT-8500 has tried to mimic this feature. Usually with imitations, the subtlety and nuance of the feature isn't as great as that of the innovator.

4. **Cervical Neck Traction**

Staying with the Inada Sogno, the airbags in the headpiece that push down onto the trapezia muscles are brilliant. Massage chairs heretofore had never been able to find a way to massage the top of the shoulders (the trapezia). Well, along comes the Sogno with its "cervical traction device," which provides airbag massage of those muscles. I love this feature, mostly because I have very tight shoulder muscles. The airbags push plastic plates with rubber nodules on them down onto the traps, and it feels like a massage therapist using elbows to massage those muscles. It is great. Osaki has tried to imitate this feature in their OS-7200H and OS-6000 models, but, again, it is not nearly as nuanced or refined as that of the Sogno.

5. **Heated Jade Rollers**

Panasonic introduced this concept into their high-end MA70 massage chair. I had seen this feature before in some massage tables by a company called Ceragem but had never seen it in a massage chair until the MA70 came out on the market. The rollers of this chair are made of jade stone, and a heating element is built in next to the stones. The heating element will warm up the stones, which in turn will provide a deep to the spinal musculature. Great idea. No one has tried to mimic this one yet.

In Part 2, I will discuss five more cool features.

10 Cool Massage Chair Features, Continued (Part 2)

In Part 1, I discussed the headband airbag massage of the Osaki OS-7075R, mechanical foot rollers, the Dreamwave technology and cervical traction device of the Inada Sogno, and the heated jade rollers of the Panasonic MA70. Here are the last five cool things you'll see when shopping for a massage chair:

6. Foot and Calf Paddles

Most chairs utilize airbags to massage the feet and calves. Airbags are OK because they provide a compression massage that can enhance circulation, but most airbags have very little motion other than direct compression. In other words, the airbags compress directly onto the muscles without much wavelike movement to enhance returning blood flow to the heart. Human Touch then came out with "paddles" in lieu of airbags. The paddles are a stiff rubberlike material that compresses in a more firm and thorough way. It actually feels like rollers massaging your calves and feet.

I had heard the term *paddles* years ago when someone at Human Touch was describing their foot and calf massage, but I didn't really know what that meant until I visited Human Touch in November and was taken on a tour of the testing area. Then I finally saw what the paddles really were…the firm rubber material. Now, if you've sat in an HT-9500x or a ZeroG 4.0, you know what I mean when I say that this technology feels like rollers. It is so much better than airbag compression; plus the paddles work in a wavelike motion to truly encourage circulation in the legs back to the heart. I absolutely love the paddle technology of the Human Touch chairs.

So if foot and calf airbags don't turn your crank too much, try out the Human Touch technology. I am sure you, too, will love it.

7. Anterior Shoulder Airbags

Shoulder airbags have come into massage chair vogue recently, but most of the airbags have been compressing the outside of the shoulders (where the deltoid muscles are located). This is OK and can also serve to pin in the user so that the rollers can seem more intense when they come up to the mid- and upper back, but the massage benefit is minimal at best. Inada came out with airbags that inflate out over the front of the shoulder joints in their Doctor's Choice 3A massage chair.

The idea behind these airbags was not to actually massage the shoulder joints but to pin the shoulders back (into a proper posture, reversing slumping shoulders). You see, it was designed to correct a slumping posture. Very cool. Well, now we see a variation of that feature in the Osaki OS-7075R and the Infinity IT-8500. You can imagine that I as a chiropractor love the posture correction aspect of this feature.

8. Thera-Elliptical Kneading

Thera-elliptical kneading was introduced by Inada in their Yume model. Whereas all other massage chairs have airbag compression (or paddle massage), the Yume offers an actual kneading motion on your calf muscles. It is pretty intense and very therapeutic. The walls of the calf wells move up and down your calves while the airbags are doing their compression thing. The result is a feeling as if someone is using their palms on your calves and massaging those muscles up and down. This is a great feature that we've not seen anywhere else.

9. Rocking

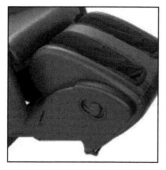

ZeroG 4.0 Ottoman

Again, Inada innovates in their Yume model with a chair that actually produces a rocking motion. It feels as if you are in a rocking chair, and it is a very soothing experience. I had one client express to me while he was sitting in the chair that it reminded him of his grandmother rocking him as a child. It was a very cathartic and even emotional experience for him. Some feel a little motion sickness the first time, but that passes very quickly.

10. Rotating Foot and Calf Ottomans

When looking for a massage chair, many people want a chair that doesn't look like a massage chair but can double as a normal-looking recliner. Not easy to do, especially with gaudy foot and calf massagers sticking out of the ottoman. Well, Human Touch innovated a retractable ottoman in their HT-1650 (now the HT-9500x) and now they have it in their Immersion Seating line (like the ZeroG 4.0). Panasonic's top-of-the-line MA70 chair has a rotating ottoman... not retracting under the seat like the Human Touch chairs but rotating under to hide the calf and footwells. The MA70 goes a long way to make their chair double as a recliner. It is a very well-engineered and well-designed chair.

This feature appeases the person who wants the massage features of the ottoman but doesn't want the ottoman to stick out like a sore thumb when it is not in use.

I hope you find these features as cool as I do. Feel free to contact me anytime if you have questions about these or any other features. I am always at your disposal.

Roller Intensity Adjustments - How?

I have spoken before about a chair's ability (or inability) to adjust the intensity of the back rollers. Most chairs have an intensity adjustment button on the remote control for the airbags in the chair, but very few have a roller intensity adjustment. For most chairs, "what you see is what you get" when it comes to the default intensity of a chair's roller system. Of course, if one person in your household or business likes a gentle massage and another likes a vigorous massage but the chair comes with a very intense default roller mechanism or vice versa, it can be tough figuring out how to get the chair to accommodate both persons' preferences.

Of the chairs we carry, these are the models that have roller intensity adjustment:

1. Inada Sogno Dreamwave

2. Human Touch HT-9500

3. HT-7450

4. HT-7120

5. ZeroG 4.0

6. Panasonic MA70

7. Panasonic EP30007

8. Panasonic EP30005

9. All Omega Montage models (Elite, Premier, Pro)

10. All Cozzia models

So how does a chair adjust for roller intensity? I didn't know until I visited Human Touch's headquarters last November and saw the inner workings and guts of many different chairs. There are two ways that I am aware of that a chair can adjust intensity:

1. Airbags

I saw on the HT-7450 and HT-9500 how airbags are located on either side of the roller mechanism. When the user increases the intensity of the rollers, the airbags deflate, thus allowing the body to lie closer to the roller mechanism. When the user decreases the intensity of the rollers, the airbags inflate to push the body away from the rollers. Very simple, but I'd never known about it or seen it before I saw it work on these two models. This method is the most common in massage chairs.

2. 3D Rollers

In chairs such as the Inada Sogno and the ZeroG 4.0, the rollers actually protrude further forward when the user increases their intensity from the remote control. And, conversely, the rollers retract when the user wants a less intense massage. This technology is becoming increasingly popular in newer massage chair models. I believe that Inada pioneered the idea.

To sit in a chair and use this function, one might never know which technology is being utilized. But as long as the intensity can be changed and you feel more comfortable while using the chair....who really cares?!

What's the Best Massage Chair for Me
if I Am Overweight?

This is a question I get asked a lot. It is a tough question to answer, particularly if you do not have the opportunity to sit in a chair and play around with it. But here are some points to consider:

1. **Weight is distributed differently** on different people. Some folks carry their extra weight around the waist, which can be a challenge in chairs that have thigh airbags. Others are just big people who carry their weight evenly distributed throughout the body. Some big folks have broad shoulders that can also prove to be a challenge in some of the chairs with shoulder airbags.

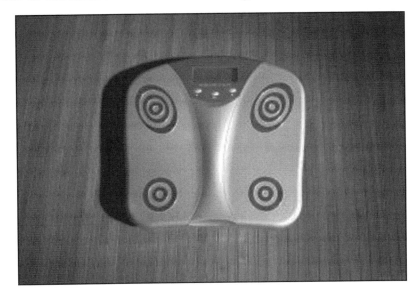

2. Massage chair companies advertise in their specs the **maximum weight for a user**. This figure is fairly nebulous, in my humble opinion, because, as I mentioned in point #1 above, weight is distributed differently in different people. If you weigh 300 pounds but are 6'5" tall, you will probably fit just fine in any chair...even if the chair states a weight limit of 265 pounds. Most chairs have a stated limited of 265 to 285 pounds.

3. You may at first feel that a chair is too small for you, but after some playing around with the chair and trying to make the fit work, you may find that you fit perfectly well. You just need to get accustomed to the chair, and you just may find the perfect position for you and your size. Here is a testimonial from a client who purchased an Inada Sogno and was quite concerned about fitting into it when he first received it (as a matter of fact, he wanted to return the chair because he didn't think he was going to fit in it at all):

Paul, New York:

Jan 29, 2012, at 10:44 AM

This review should help people who are big in size and weight and are on the fence to jump off and make the purchase!

I am a 5 feet 11 inch, 315 pound, 40-year-old man who suffers from an incurable medical condition that bombards me with chronic pain.

I had an issue trying to sit on the chair without breaking and crushing the hip airbags. I thought I wasn't going to be able to use this wonderful therapeutic relaxing healing machine...but after trying over and over, I gave up on it and was going to return it....Then I decided NOT to give up and try again....Success!!! I was able to negotiate safely and properly a way to get into the chair without crushing the hip airbags. Once in, everything was perfect!

First off, Inada should rename its proprietary Dreamwave to Goodnight Irene because this feature will make you want to sleep in no time. It rocks and sways your seat, hips, and hip and leg muscles in a way that you've just got to try. It's like floating on a wave and being stretched and held in a god's arms. Every preset massage program is amazing as the chair reads your Shiatsu points and length and width of your spine....The stretch program is one of my favorites....Awwww heck, they're all my favorites.

On the bottom of the easy-to-use remote are the manual commands so you can designate a certain part of the body to concentrate only on. The heat controls are a nice touch, and the ottoman will make your feet and calves feel like a million bucks. There's also a metal plate with half-moon balls on it that pushes up and massages the bottom of your feet...wonderful!!

You can use the strength of the airbags and rollers with the default settings out of the box, or you can adjust the strength and pressure with the remote if you find it too hard for you...but remember, if you have tight, unused muscles or knots everywhere, this machine will take care of them, but if you feel that it hurts, it's because you're not used to massages and manipulation of blood and muscles. This is a truly remarkable machine....Give it time....You will want to put this machine in your will...lol.

At 315 pounds, while in the chair, the motor spoke to me....It said, "Paul, relax. I'm an Inada. If you can fit, you can sit. Now, relax and enjoy the massage. I can hold your weight with no problem." You will find it hard to believe that there aren't human hands inside this machine! Stress and pain melt away.

Price, yeah, I know it's expensive; however, it's WORTH EVERY CENT!!!!!! This is no Chinese inferior-made product. This is no cheap mall outlet chair with a cheesy 90-day to a measly one-year warranty. This isn't a chair manufactured by some fly-by-night company that doesn't back up their product 100%.

Now, Dr. Weidner, a patient and super-informative expert on massage chairs, will guide you with a no-pressure experience. Although I just received my chair, I know if there's anything I need or if I have any questions, he will be there before and after the sale. The very same goes for InadaUSA. Nice folks.

So if you're big like me or not, you simply CANNOT purchase a better massage chair, and you cannot get an upper-echelon manufactured massage chair for under $4K. This price point for this chair fits the bill for its therapeutic capability and excellence in manufacturing....Folks, there is a HUGE and noticeable difference in the make and performance of this beautifully designed machine.

I purchased mine in dark brown....WARNING....when it's not in the right light, it looks pure black....Even my delivery guys thought it was black....It's a TRUE dark brown, and it's a stunning addition to anybody's home.

The reason I wanted to rush and hurry up my review for this chair is so that anybody who is considering it to NOT wait till Feb. 1st when this chair increases in price $800. Be a smart and savvy consumer and make this call to Dr. Weidner and staff!!!!

I hope this helped people who are overweight and/or hesitant, and I hope this helped out people who need to know this chair's almost infinite capabilities...but...you need to sit in it first.

Of course, I can't explain every feature and nook and cranny unless you're in the mood to read a short novel...lol!!

Thank you for reading my review on the Inada Dreamwave Plus massage chair.

P.S. I am 310 lbs currently, been dieting for two weeks...just weighed myself while writing this...-5 pounds....I'll take it. I forgot, when you get off the chair, you will notice improved circulation, better breathing, well-being, happiness, feeling alive, more energy, and the body's natural pain blockers in full effect!!

Awesome!

4. One thing that a number of clients have done prior to purchasing a chair from me is have me give them **measurements of the seat width between the two chair sides** and tell them whether those sides are restricted by the built-in armrests or thigh airbags. Some chairs are definitely wider than others. Typically, chairs without the thigh airbags—such as the HT-7120 or HT-7450, for example—have a wider berth than a chair such as the Panasonic 30007 or the IT-8200/IT-8500. You can measure your seat width in a seated position and then compare it to the seat width of the chair you are interested in. Now, let me just say that this is not a guarantee that the chair will or will not work for you. I have seen what seemed to be narrow seat widths work just fine for a larger waistline. By the way, this applies to shoulder widths and shoulder airbag restrictions as well as seats and thigh airbags.

I am always available to get that seat or shoulder measurement on any chair I carry. Just give me a call, and I'll see what I can do to get you into the right chair.

Sleeping in a Massage Chair?

A question I frequently get from massage chair shoppers is what chair would be best suited for sleeping...that is sleeping *in*? Now, I must confess I have fallen asleep in many a massage chair in my day, and the word Sogno actually means *dream* (I am referring to the famous Inada Sogno Dreamwave massage chair), but to sleep the night away in a massage chair doesn't seem all that comfortable to me.

Having said that, there are folks out there—and you may be one of them—who have terrible back or neck pain who can't lie flat on a conventional bed. Someone may be recovering from surgery and can't lie flat on his or her back or on his or her side. There are also people who snore and have sleep apnea who can sleep only in an inclined position. So it totally makes sense that somebody might want a massage chair that is comfortable for sleeping.

Here are things to consider when deciding on what type of massage chair would be best suited for sleeping:

1. **Calf and foot massage mechanism** – This is probably the single greatest inhibitor of comfort for someone who wants to sleep in a massage chair. You can't really put your legs anywhere else besides the calf and footwells. If you move to your side on the chair, your legs will still tend to relocate to the calf wells. If you want to shift your body while on your back, your legs won't really be able to move anywhere because their movement is limited by the width of the calf wells and footwells.

An answer to this issue might be a chair that has a rotating otto-man so that the calf wells and footwells can be rotated out of the way. An example of this might be the Panasonic MA70, which has a foot and calf ottoman that rotates under and looks like a normal ottoman on which legs can be moved anywhere. Another option might be the HT-7450 or HT-7120 chairs by Human Touch. They have only calf wells so that the ottoman can be easily rotated upside down, allowing for a flat ottoman surface on which the legs can be moved wherever the user wants to put them.

2. **Rollers** – When the chair is off and at rest, where are the rollers? If they are *parked*, which means that they are retracted so that they don't stick out, you can sit in the chair and not really feel them at all. If a chair doesn't park the rollers, they may be sticking out at rest and actually stick into your back. Not very comfortable.

Another thing to consider regarding the rollers is the roller track space that is vacated when the rollers themselves are retracted and parked. When you sit in a massage chair without the rollers on, your back kind of sinks into the roller space, and that is not optimal sup-port for the low back. You may need to put a pillow in the low back/lumbar region to support your low back or else you may wake up in more pain than when you went to sleep.

3. **Sleeping on your side** – Massage chairs are not really built for side sleeping or lying. It will be difficult to find a place to put your legs (unless the chair has a rotating ottoman—see #1 above) and you will not have a lot of room to curl up, which is a common position to sleep in when on your side. I think the hardness of the chair may also contribute to spot tenderness on your body when you sleep on your side. Make sure the chair reclines back to at least 170 degrees or more, which is close to horizontal, so that your body is not bent up from sleeping on your side.

Well, that's about it for sleeping considerations when getting a massage chair. I also might mention that all massage chair companies that I am aware of have time limits for their massage sessions. I think one of the reasons for that is if the user falls asleep. If a deep sleeper sits in the chair and the timer were to never turn off, that poor soul may be so sore in the morning from an all-nighter in a massage chair that he or she may never sit on it again. Yes, too much of a good thing is not always a good thing.

No-Name Brand Chairs – My Thoughts

I get a call probably once a week from a massage chair shopper or owner asking about some no-name brand massage chair. Either he or she wants to know if I've heard of the brand or if I know how the owner can get some customer support for a broken-down chair from a company whose phone number is no longer in service.

Well, here is a question like that from a massage chair shopper. I thought I should post this one because the situation is very common and scary!!

Question:

I have been looking for a chair for six months. Of course, the Inada may be the best but is too high for my budget. The Infinity IT8200 would be good for me at 3,195.00 with a free IT2020 neck massager. However, I found a look-alike BeautyHealth chair for 1,999.00, with a 10-year warranty, but this scares me. I have learned that what seems to be too good to be true usually is. Who can I trust on the Internet to stand behind my $2,000.00 to $3,500.00 purchase? I can get a six-month-old floor model Inada for around $5,500 including tax, but that is a little more than my budget. I do like the hand control of the Inada. The Infinity control looks a little complicated to me. I saw you talking about the chairs on the Internet, and I think that you would stand behind what you sell. Do you know anything about the BeautyHealth chairs?

My Answer:

Hi, Len.

Thank you so much for your e-mail and trusting me enough to ask my opinion.

My first suggestion would be to run away from any chair that offers a ten-year warranty! No reputable company offers that, and I just might add that I have had calls from BeautyHealth customers very upset that they cannot get satisfactory customer support. What good is a warranty if you can't get a hold of any customer support folks when a problem arises with your chair? Your comment that it is probably too good to be true is no truer than when it applies to massage chairs. My strong recommendation would be to stick with a name brand.

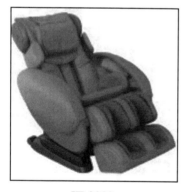

IT-8200

Infinite Therapeutics, though a smaller player in the massage chair market, is a very good company with great customer support. You will be fine going with them for your massage chair. The IT-8200 is a very nice chair. We recently got it in our showroom, and from early responses, our clients seem to really like it. It is an Inada Sogno look-alike. Looking like the Sogno is where the comparison ends. The Inada chairs are phenomenal, and that is reflected in the price.

The foot rollers in the IT-8200 are fantastic. I really enjoy that feature. I think you would, too. The remote control on the IT-8200 is a pedestal remote as you can tell from the pictures, but it is remarkably easy to use. It is a touch screen, and I did not find the controls intimidating at all. I have felt intimidated by massage chair remote controls in the past, like with the Sanyo 7700 and the Panasonic 30007, but this one was very easy to get comfortable with.

Yes, I do certainly stand behind what I sell. I might also mention that I don't sell chairs that don't have a good customer support record. If you ever have a problem with your chair, I want you to be able to feel secure in knowing that you have full support behind you. And should you ever have a problem with a chair and are having trouble with getting a hold of the company, give me a call and I will get involved to make sure that you are taken care of. Lousy customer service by a massage chair company reflects on me and my retail business...and, personally, I can't stand that.

In that same price range of $2,000–$3,500 you might also check out some Osaki chairs. They are also Chinese chairs like the IT-8200 and have become very popular. They have a good customer support department, and like the IT-8200, you get a pretty good bang for your buck.

Shipping Massage Chairs to Canada

(or any country for that matter!)

I have been getting a lot of calls from prospective massage chair shoppers in Canada. The US dollar (USD) must be getting a little stronger lately. Our family just got back from our annual pilgrimage to Canada (the birthplace of both my wife and I and three of our six children), and when I reviewed my debit card statement upon coming back to Utah, I saw that the exchange rate favored the US. I was a bit surprised by that since the USD had gotten so weak that the Canadian dollar was stronger than ours just a few short months ago.

Usually when I start getting more international inquiries, that is a pretty good indication that the currency in another country is dropping in value.

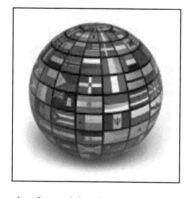

Well, I figured I'd write a brief blog post about shipping to Canada since I've been getting the same questions more frequently as of late. For most of our massage chairs, free shipping still applies to Canada. If you live somewhere "way up north," such as Fort McMurray or into the Yukon or NWT, the shipping will be more. But for major cities and business centers, the free shipping usually applies. Just call me to make sure.

The only holdup and logistical issue that needs addressing is customs. When you are importing a massage chair from the US, you will need to pay customs/duty tax. I am not sure how much it is, but it is probably comparable to the current GST rate. Don't take my word for it, though. Call a customs broker to be sure.

Now, here is what you have to do when you order a massage chair from the USA:

Contact a customs broker! They are businesses that will process your chair paperwork into Canada by working through the customs duty/tax fees. You *must* go through a customs broker. The rule is that the owner of the chair has to make that arrangement. I can't do it for you because I am just the facilitator of the sale. You will need to contact a customs broker to make arrangements for duty. Here is one that my shippers recommend:

YRC Customs Brokerage (866)568-5588

Here is how it works:

1. Buyer needs to contact and sign up with a customs broker (small fee required).

2. Buyer passes along customs broker contact info to Massage-Chair-Relief.com.

3. We pass the customs broker contact info to our shipping broker.

4. Shipping broker passes contact info to the driver of the truck carrying your new massage chair.

5. When the truck hits the border, the driver will contact the customs broker and complete the process to get the chair into the country.

6. The shipping company will contact you to make arrangements for a convenient delivery time to your home or business.

I hope this helps those of you who are Canadian residents looking to get a massage chair from the US. These basic customs principles apply to any international shipment, but logistics can be different, i.e., ocean vs. air freight vs. land freight, protocol for paying the customs duty/tax, etc.

Zero Gravity vs. Inversion

In the past, I have written about zero gravity to dispel misconceptions about what it really is.

http://www.massage-chair-relief.com/blog/chair-models/zero-gravity-massage-chairs/

Every massage chair seems to be using the zero-gravity feature, and it has become very popular. But the inversion feature is fairly new to the industry, and most folks think that it is the same thing as zero gravity. It is actually quite different.

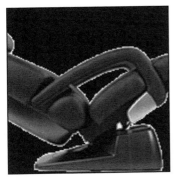

Zero Gravity

While zero gravity is nothing more than a 30-degree tilt of the massage chair seat, inversion is actually reclining the chair back to below horizontal so that the body becomes somewhat inverted.

You may be familiar with inversion therapy from TV commercials or from a chiropractic office. To invert means "to turn upside down." An inversion machine is designed to turn the user upside down so that his or her head is down and the feet are up. The idea is to invert so that the spine is being stretched or elongated with the notion that inversion will relieve back pain. Users buckle up their ankles so that when they turn themselves upside down, the body stays inverted and doesn't fall to the ground.

When I practiced chiropractic, I had many patients who told me that they had used an inversion machine. For some it helped; for some it didn't. At that time, there was no real research to back inversion up or not, but from the stories many patients told me, it seemed to do a lot of good.

Inversion was introduced in the not-too-distant past to massage chairs to try mimicking that therapeutic effect. The best the massage chair can do to that end is recline the chair back past the horizontal position of 180 degrees. Once it passes that point, gravity begins to serve as a source of distraction on the spine. When you sit in the chair, you can actually feel as though you are going past horizontal, and you actually feel as though you are going to slide off the chair back. (By the way, some zero-gravity chairs that don't have inversion give you the feeling that you are going to slide off the chair back when the chair is reclined in the zero-gravity position. The HT-7450 is an example.)

Does inversion have any therapeutic effect? I don't know, but folks seem to like it. Is it as effective as a real inversion machine? Unlikely, but at least it offers some degree of inversion. I suppose that any-thing is better than nothing in this situation.

There are currently two chairs that we carry that offer inversion:

1) IT-9800 – The specs show that the chair back reclines to 183 degrees.

2) IT-8500 – Infinite Therapeutics touts this chair as an inversion chair, but its specs show the recline to be only 178 degrees, which seems to me to be higher than the horizontal of 180 degrees.

Is inversion the next massage chair fad like zero gravity is now? Well, we shall see.

I hope to have both these models in my showroom before the end of summer. I will gladly review and videotape them for your perusal at that time.

Massage Chair Airbags – Helpful or a Waste of Air?

When the massage chair was first introduced to the market in 1962, it was Mr. Inada's basic invention of rollers going up and down the spine. The concept of airbags did not come for some time after that. Nowadays, we see airbags in more parts of the body of the chair than there are rollers. For example, in some of the more feature-rich massage chairs, you will see airbags in the following places:

1. Feet and calves

2. Buttock

3. Thigh

4. Waist

5. Shoulders – front, back, side, and rear!

6. Arms and hands

7. Trapezia muscles

8. Neck

9. Head (The new Osaki 7000 massage chair actually has a head-band that you put around your skull that has airbags that massage your skull and suboccipital muscles…ideal for stress headache sufferers.)

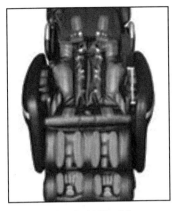

Osaki OS-6000 airbags

I'm sure there will be even more places that the manufacturing companies think of to put an airbag. Who knows? They may even be testing airbags for the front of your body for all I know.

Well, I guess the big question that I get from massage chair shoppers regarding airbags is not "How many airbags does this or that massage chair have?", but "Do airbags really do anything?"

Great question, and here is my input on that query. The primary function of airbags is to compress a body part. In some cases, such as in the Inada Sogno Dreamwave, airbags actually serve to also move the seat, which induces passive motion to the pelvis and low back—a wonderful feature that is unique to that model. But for all the rest of the airbags, I can't think of any other purpose than to compress body parts.

If you've tried out a massage chair, you've probably experienced the foot and calf massage. This is typically the most popular and commonly seen airbag set on most chairs. You felt the compression on your calves and feet. For some of you, the compression was too much and too intense. For others, it was not enough or just right. Well, imagine having circulation problems. For poor circulation, many folks experience swelling of the feet and ankles. And what is the typical home treatment for that? Compression hosiery/socks. Can you see how the airbags of a massage chair can mimic that compression, not just passively as with socks but actively with motion of the airbags starting from the feet and moving upward in a wavelike manner toward the heart?

Now, if it is helpful for swollen ankles, which we see that it is, can you see how it may serve a normal foot and ankle just by enhancing circulation back to the heart? In this case, I believe that the airbag compression encourages healthy circulation from foot to heart. I suppose the same could be said for hand and arm airbag compression since these components also "milk" the body part toward the heart.

Massage Chair Airbags Do More than Just Compress…

Some airbags compress not to improve circulation but to move a body part in a particular direction. For example, we are seeing many massage chairs come into the market now that have waist airbags that push one side of the low back forward and then the other. Simultaneous to that, the airbags of the seat may inflate on one side or the other to induce a rotation of the low back. You see, on one side, the waist airbag is inflated while on the other side the seat airbag is inflated. This induces rotation to the low back, which in the past has been a difficult motion to reproduce passively in a massage chair. I have felt that rotation in many of the massage chairs in my showroom, and it is actually fantastic and appears to have a real therapeutic benefit for the soft tissues of the low back.

Now, as far as the other airbags go, I suppose it is truly a personal preference. An airbag in some body location may be just what you need to overcome some pain or other distress. What may work for one may not affect another the same way. I have heard from clients who thought that the shoulder airbag massage of the Inada Sogno or Osaki 6000 was the answer to a chronic trapezius muscle tightness. But others didn't think it did anything but annoy them. So as the Spanish would say, "*Cada cabeza es un mundo*," or in plain English, "to each his own."

When Exactly Does a Massage Chair Warranty Begin??

I get this question a lot, and to be frank, I have always just said, "When the chair ships out." That sounds pretty good, and most folks believed it…heck, I believed it. Well, I was discussing a **massage chair** purchase with a customer on the phone yesterday, and the subject came up again.

This time, doggone it, I really wanted to know. I actually don't like just saying stuff to satisfy a client if I myself am not sure of the answer. So I took it upon myself this morning to contact all of my massage chair manufacturer reps and find out exactly what the policy is regarding when the warranty kicks in.

Is it when the chair is purchased by the client? Is it when I place the order with the massage chair company? Is it when the chair ships? How about when it delivers? Of course, this only really matters if a problem arises the week that the warranty is supposed to expire. Otherwise, a week or two won't make that big of a difference. But what happens if this scenario plays out…one year and two days after the client has purchased his or her massage chair, the warranty expires, and something goes wrong with the chair. Will the massage chair company honor the warranty from the date of delivery to the home or business of the client? Well, here are the answers for each of the companies for which I sell massage chairs:

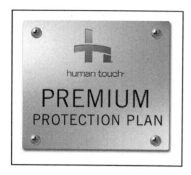

1. **Human Touch** – The company policy is that the warranty begins when the chair is purchased by the end user. So I asked what happens if the order is placed and the chair is back-ordered for a week or month...or more! I was told by the customer support rep at Human Touch that the company is flexible in situations like that. If it comes to a situation like that, Human Touch will consider the delivery date as the beginning point of the warranty. Remember, this is not in writing as company policy, but it seems to be a general rule of thumb for customer support folks at Human Touch.

2. **Inada** – The purchase date of an Inada massage chair is considered the beginning of the warranty, but speaking with Inada directly, I was told that should a problem arise during that critical end-of-warranty period, Inada will check the proof of delivery date and go with that date. No fuss, no muss.

3. **Osaki** – Osaki considers the delivery date to the client's home or business as the beginning of the warranty period.

4. **Infinite Therapeutics** – Like Osaki, the company policy for IT chairs also considers the delivery date as the beginning of the warranty period.

5. **Panasonic and Sanyo** – Same company now, so very similar policies. The purchase date is considered the beginning of the warranty, but should a situation arise as I described above, Panasonic and Sanyo will side with the delivery date as the warranty beginning.

You know, come to think of it, it might not be a bad idea at all to save the receipt from the shipping company on the day of your massage chair delivery. You just might need it one, two, three, or five years down the road if a problem arises on the anniversary of your warranty.

6. **Omega** – Date of purchase. Now, Omega was the only company that didn't get back to me, so I can't speak for them about using the delivery date as the warranty beginning. But they are good folks over there, so I would assume that would be the case. When I hear from them, I will share that info in this blog with an update.

By the way, if your massage chair comes with a warranty registration card, *please make sure* that you fill it out and send it back to the massage chair company. For some companies, such as Omega, the policy is "no warranty registration card, no warranty." So, just like saving the delivery receipt, make sure to send in the warranty registration card if there is one with the massage chair you purchased.

Stretch Programs in Massage Chairs

The term *stretch* has a totally different meaning to me as a chiropractor than it does in the **massage chair** industry.

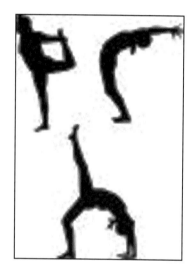

When I was a practicing chiropractor, we found that lots and lots of patients had imbalanced muscle groups. Some muscles were too tight, and others were too weak. I spent an awful lot of my time coaching patients with stretching and strengthening regimens. Of course, the stretching was for tight muscles, and the strengthening was for weak muscles.

For example, when a person had low back pain, almost in every case, that person had tight hamstrings and hip flexors along with weak abdominals and gluteals. So our treatment always included stretching those muscles groups in the clinic and then teaching the patient how to do it at home.

When patients followed the home exercise protocols that I prescribed, they almost always felt better and were pain-free in a fairly short period of time.

Stretch Done by a Massage Chair? No Way!

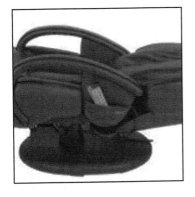

Well, then I got into the massage chair business. The first chair I ever owned and used in my clinic was the Human Touch HT-125, a very basic but durable massage chair. I noticed that it had a program on it called Stretch. I thought, "Holy mackerel, how on earth did this company incorporate stretching into a massage chair, and what muscles does this chair stretch?"

A few patients had told me how much they loved the stretch program. I had not used that program to that point (most massage chairs come with many different automatic programs, and I always use the Full Body program, if there is one, so that I get a good once-over in a short period of time). I figured I'd better give this stretch program a shot.

It turned out to be nothing like what I had expected or what I had been clinically trained for in my profession.

This is what I experienced: The chair reclined to 170 degrees (almost completely horizontal), and the ottoman came up to a horizontal position. At that point, the airbags inflated around my calves and held them tightly. Once that happened, the ottoman went down, thus tractioning my whole body, and the rollers started to roll up and down my spine.

It was a little uncomfortable at first because my body was not used to being put in an arched position, which is how it felt. It seemed to hyperextend my back. Now, I already have a lumbar (low back) spine curvature that is exaggerated, so the arching isn't best for my type of spine. But for those clients who have a normal or decreased lumbar curve, the stretch function is awesome.

Oh, So That's What They Meant by a Massage Chair Stretch!

So, regarding the HT-125, the stretching is more of an arching and tractioning of the spine.

When I began carrying other massage chairs, such as the Inada Sogno and the Panasonic 30007, I noticed that they, too, had stretch programs. But when I tried out their programs, they were nothing like that of the Human Touch HT-125 massage chair.

The stretch programs in these chairs were more of a gentle "milking," as I like to call it, of the spine and discs. The ottomans went up and down while the chair backs alternately reclined and inclined. It was a very lovely feeling to have that going on with my spine. I actually loved the way it felt but, again, very different from the HT-125 massage chair.

It really is a very personal preference, but it seems as though the stretch program is a popular one and will most likely be on many future massage chair models for years to come. I cannot recall one person ever coming to our massage chair showroom and not enjoying the stretch program on at least one massage chair. And in many cases, it was one of their favorite programs.

b) Massage Chair Glossary

In your search for the perfect massage chair, you have probably come across terms or words that you have never heard of before. You may even think you want a particular feature because everyone talks about it, yet you don't really even know what it means. I know I experienced that quite a bit when I first got into this business.

I created this glossary for customers just like you who may need a little explanation when it comes to certain terms that we in the massage chair business use every single day without even thinking about them.

1. **Zero gravity** – In the massage chair business, *zero gravity* refers to the positioning of the chair when the seat is tilted at a 30-degree angle, and the chair back and seat articulate with each other at a 120-degree angle. This was deemed by NASA to be the most stress-free position for astronauts in a seated position. Massage chair companies have integrated this technology into their products. You will feel that less stress is placed on the low back when zero-gravity positioning is engaged.

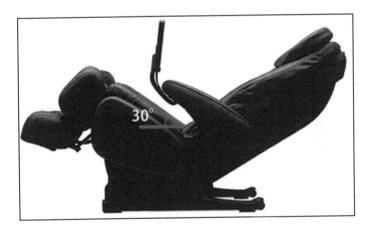

Zero-gravity positioning

2. **Roller track** – The roller track is the housing for the rollers that perform the massage functions on the spine of the user. The rollers move on this roller track to extend from the top to the bottom of the track.

Many manufacturers and retailers refer to the *massage stroke length*. This essentially is the length of the roller track. Most tracks are 26–31 inches long, but newer models now extend to almost 50 inches in length.

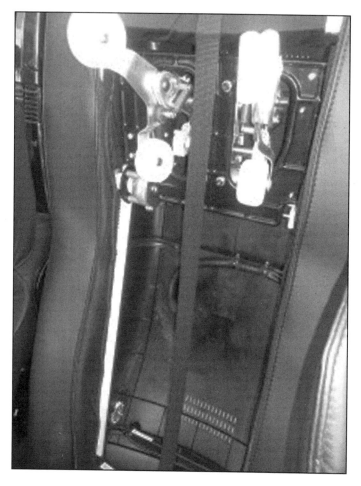

Roller track

3. **S-shape roller track** – From a side view, the shape of your spine is not straight but made up of a series of forward and backward curves...the neck (cervical) and low back (lumbar) have forward curves; the midback (thoracic) and pelvis have backward curves.

This sinuous shape of the spine is referred to in the massage chair industry as *S-shape*. Most chairs have roller tracks that are S-shaped in order to conform to the natural shape of your spine.

In the early days of this industry, the first massage chairs had straight roller tracks, which did not conform to the shape of the human spine; thus, some areas did not get as effective a massage as others. The introduction of the S-shape roller track made it possible for every segment of your spine to get a good massage from the rollers.

3. **Quad rollers** – Most chairs nowadays have four rollers that move up and down the roller track—two on each side. These rollers are usually arranged so that the top two rollers protrude farther forward than the bottom two rollers. This design was created to accommodate the changing curvature of the spine…when the curve changes, the upper two rollers will hit the coming curve, while the bottom two rollers will still be set back enough to hit the previous curve.

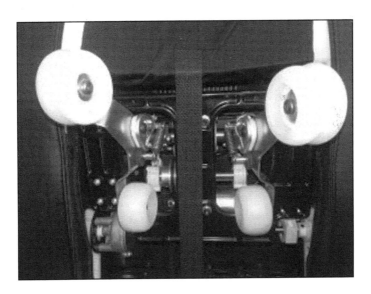

4. **3D rollers** – All rollers move from side to side and up and down, which represent the x and y axes of movement, respectively. Until recently, very few rollers actually moved forward and back, which

is movement along the z axis. Previously, only two dimensions of motion were offered by roller systems. Now, chairs are coming out with the z axis dimension of motion—movement forward and back—which provides the ability to increase or decrease the intensity of the roller massage.

5. **Kneading** – Every massage chair has its own proprietary technology to perform basic massage functions. Kneading is one of those functions. It usually involves the rollers working in a small circular motion while at the same time moving toward and away from the spine.

6. **Shiatsu** – The word *Shiatsu* means *finger pressure*. When I was a practicing chiropractor, I often performed *trigger point therapy*, in which we would apply specific pressure to a muscle with the intent of getting it to relax. Shiatsu can be thought of as a form of trigger point pressure. The Shiatsu function on a massage chair typically involves the rollers hitting a spot and staying on it for a few seconds to apply a fingerlike pressure. Some chairs will also move the rollers in a very, very tight circle while pressing against the muscle. It can be uncomfortable for some, but it is a very therapeutic mode in a massage chair.

7. **Airbags** – Airbags can be defined in two ways: as airbags or air cells within an airbag. Airbags have become very common on most massage chairs. They are used for things such as arm or leg compression, moving the chair seat, neck and shoulder massage, waist and seat pressure, moving the rollers forward and back, and much more. They are literally airbags that inflate via a compressor in the chair. An airbag can be just one airbag or can contain multiple air cells that work together to effect a total airbag massage.

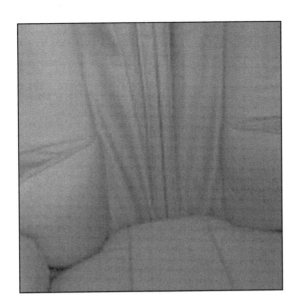

Waist airbags

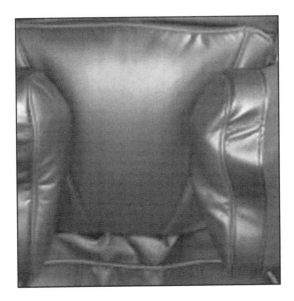

Thigh airbags

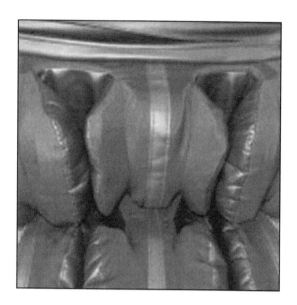

Calf and feet airbags

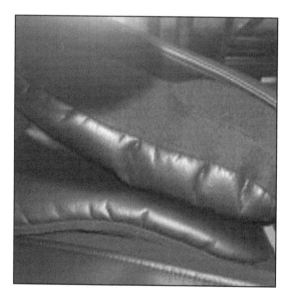

Arm airbags

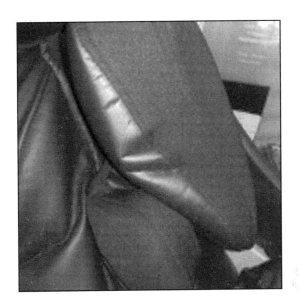

Upper arm airbags

8. **Inversion** – True inversion involves turning the body upside down, or at least past horizontal, to decompress the spine. Many of my patients have used inversion tables at home for back pain relief. The definition of inversion as it relates to massage chairs is that if the chair back reclines past 180 degrees (horizontal), then it is inverting and thus the spine is decompressing to some degree. There are not many chairs that have a true inversion feature, but some come awfully close to a horizontal recline. If you come across a chair that touts an inversion feature, double-check to make sure it truly has a reclining angle of greater than 180 degrees.

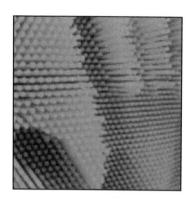

9. Body scan technology – Scanning has become a standard feature in most massage chairs. The idea behind body scantechnology is that the chair scans the body before beginning a massage to make sure that the program caters to the body shape and size of the user. Some scanning technologies are very sophisticated (i.e., Inada) where the chair has a series of infrared lights that outline the shape of your spine. It then matches that outline to a database of over 150 spinal shapes, finding the spinal shape closest to yours.

Other chairs use a very simple scanning technology that only finds out where your head and shoulders are so that the rollers don't travel too high up your back and onto your skull. That does not feel very good, FYI! It is important to keep your head back during a body scan so that the chair can truly determine where it needs to send its rollers.

10. Mechanical foot rollers – Airbags compressing the calves and feet are commonplace in the massage chair industry, but now chairs are coming out with mini-rollers under your feet that rotate and massage the soles of your feet. It is a novel idea that a lot of folks are latching onto. It can become a bit overbearing after a few minutes if you are not used to having your feet massaged or even touched. Combined with the feet airbags, the rollers offer really good therapy.

11. **Dreamwave** – Inada coined this phrase for their Sogno model. It is a program that utilizes an airbag technology in the seat to move the seat from side to side in a figure-eight motion while also lifting the seat up and down. It is a great feature for soothing the low back musculature, particularly for acute low back pain.

12. **Retractable ottoman** – The ottoman houses the foot- and calf-massaging mechanisms. A few models allow for the user to hide the calf wells and footwells by having an ottoman that can either be rotated or retracted. The rotation feature allows you to spin the ottoman around, leaving a flat surface to face the room. The retractable ottoman actually gets pulled into the chair and under the seat to completely obscure the ottoman from view.

This is a great feature for someone who wants a massage chair for its function but not for its looks...who would rather have the chair look like a regular recliner than a therapeutic machine. <u>Human Touch</u> has been the industry leader in obscuring ottomans from view.

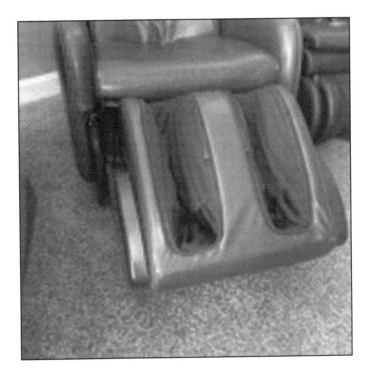

Ottoman out

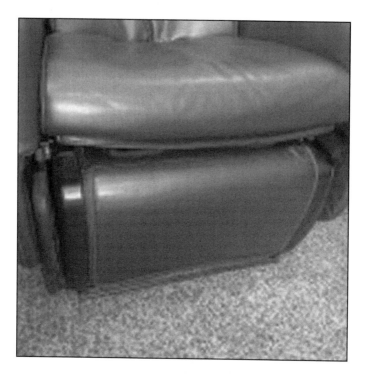

Ottoman retracted

13. **Stretch program** – When you think of stretching, you probably envision a hamstring or quadriceps stretch, or bending over to touch your toes. Well, no chairs can do that...yet, anyway. But what they can do is use the chair back, the ottoman, the shoulder and feet airbags, and the roller system to distract (pull) the body or arch the body.

The most common stretch program has airbags grabbing the feet and ankles in the ottoman, as well as shoulder airbags pinning the shoulders back. The chair back and ottoman rise up and lower down to put the body into an arched position. Many chairs then use the rollers to go down into the low back, which accentuates the arch even more.

This is a typical stretch program. Other chairs add little things to change it up somewhat, such as pulling the arms or legs away from the body or bringing the ottoman and chair back up as high as possible to induce flexion of the body. Every manufacturer seems to have a little twist here and there for each of their models to make it a little different.

I hope this has assisted you in becoming more familiar with what the terms in the massage chair business actually mean.

c) Reviews and Testimonials

Here are just a few of the very satisfied testimonials I've collected from "patients" around the world who have purchased a robotic massage chair at Massage-Chair-Relief.com (you can visit http://www.massage-chair-relief.com/clients_speak.html for a bunch of testimonials from our clients. You can also go to **any product page on our site** and read reviews left by our customers about their experience with their chair and our company.

"I really appreciate the before-delivery e-mails from you."

Thanks, Alan.

I received the massage chair on Saturday within the shipping period you stated. The shipping company was excellent; the individual who delivered the chair to my home was not only professional but very nice! I have already used and set up the chair with no problems. By the way, I really appreciate the before-delivery e-mails from you; it was a nice way of keeping me on track of the different stages of the delivery. Much thanks,

Stan Tolan
Gardena, California

"Your price matching, which was incredibly easy and totally in line with your claims, helped out."

Thanks for your great service getting us our chair. We purchased the Omega Ion chair, and we LOVE it. My wife has chronic back and neck problems so her doctor recommended we purchase a massage chair. Without being rich, we were worried about the expense. But your price matching, which was incredibly easy and totally in line with your claims, helped out. The chair was delivered a week earlier than expected, and our backs are so thankful. My wife uses it every day, and it is making a real difference. The only problem is keeping our friends from coming over at all hours to lounge in it. Thanks for the service and the great product. We're thrilled! Thanks,

Tim and Ginny Thompson
Madison, WI

"We would recommend Massage Chair Relief to anyone who is interested in buying a massage chair."

When we first came to the store in Salt Lake, it was awesome. Stephanie was so nice and knowledgeable about all the chairs that were in the showroom. She had us take off our shoes and sit in each chair to see the differences between the chairs. We left that day very happy and discussing which chairs we liked the most. The next day, we went to another store here and were very disappointed in the customer service and selection that was available. So we went back to Massage Chair Relief. We spent nine hours in the store that day. We left for dinner and returned to buy two chairs. They were so helpful and friendly. When our chairs were delivered, it was a week later. We were so excited that we called our family to come and sit in the chairs. After my father-in-law sat in my chair, he went to the store and got his own. We would recommend Massage Chair Relief to anyone who is interested in buying a massage chair. If you live in

Utah or surrounding states, make the trip to the store. It will be well worth it. Thank you, Dr. Al and Stephanie. We love you guys, and we love our chairs.

**David and Brook Gonzales
Sandy, Utah**

"Customer service was especially surprising.... You have been great to deal with."

Dear Dr. Weidner,

Thank you for offering the massage chair at an affordable price to your patients. It has been an important investment in our health. We knew the value of the chair because we had already tried one in a specialty store. It was an easy decision to make.

I have an ongoing problem with my neck, shoulders, and lower back, and our chair has proven to be a great way to relieve stress and pain from my neck and spine. I am very glad we purchased it and use it on a regular basis, almost every day.

Customer service was especially surprising, also. During shipment, our chair was slightly torn. They were so helpful and nice on the phone, and within a short period of time, the company delivered a complete new chair to our door and brought it in, unpacked it for us, and took the damaged one.

Thank you again, Dr. Weidner, for a pleasant and beneficial experience, both by the company, and from you. You have been especially great to deal with.

Marilyn Broadhead

"It is a pleasure to buy from http://www.massage-chair-relief.coml."

I ordered this chair for my husband as a gift. It is a pleasure to buy from http://www.massage-chair-relief.com/ and has very good communication. Highly Recommended.

The chair was a snap to set up. The controls are easy to use, and the many different massage options hit about every spot on the body—including feet! The leather is nice and soft; it looks beautiful in my family room. Thank you,

Susan Qiu
Texas

"I was scared ordering a big purchase item through a website, but rest assured, these guys...are trustworthy."

I bought a Sanyo massage chair from this website through a price match, and they had the BEST deal with extra bonus gifts and EXCELLENT customer service when I called them through the phone. I was scared ordering a big purchase item through a website, but rest assured, these guys answered my questions and are trustworthy. Pleasure doing business with them; the chair is working great. Thanks.

Varinder Singh
Hicksville, NY

"My husband...is telling all the guys he works with to come and get a chair from you!"

I just have to share one thing with you—I have been trying to get my husband to look at those chairs since Christmas. I wanted to get one for him for Christmas, and he wouldn't do it. So it was his birthday and Father's Day, and I told him I wanted to get a chair for him. He was very hesitant when I brought him in there. Anyway, he has back and leg issues, and he now has used the chair three times—and I just talked to him—he works for (company withheld)—and he is telling all the guys he works with to come and get a chair from you. He said they work. He is a great spokesman for your chairs! So—he is sending people in there—some of the guys are under the impression they just vibrate. He told them it is a full-blown massage—and it works. He made my day—and I want to thank you guys. Please tell Dr. Weidner that I said thank you. Watch for the boys from (company withheld). Thank you so much!!

Bonnie Higgins
Salt Lake City, Utah

"It has truly improved our quality of life!"

Hi, Dr. Weidner,

Just wanted to let you know that we are definitely loving our new chair. I apologize for not writing sooner, but we also just started about five new daily therapies for our autistic son, so when we haven't been doing that, we've been IN the chair! The Inada is everything for which I hoped and more. The customer service was excellent, the chair was easy to operate, and all I do is tell my friends how fantastic this chair has been for us and how it has been worth every penny.

I've even started getting a "Chair Massage Day" playgroup going for moms of other autistic children, because if anyone deserves a weekly half hour in this wonderfully relaxing massage chair, it's parents with special-needs kids!

Overall, we couldn't be more pleased with EVERYTHING about this amazing chair. You were absolutely right that I would love it. I could go on and on about how therapeutic it has been for all of us. We have improved relaxation, improved energy, more patience—it has truly improved our quality of life, and how often can you say that about a piece of furniture?!

Many thanks again for all your outstanding customer service, Dr. Weidner!

All the best,

Dawn Hardy
Metairie, Louisianna

"No wonder you have a AAA rating from BBB.org."

This chair is a gift for my father, and he loves his new chair. My buying process was easy, and you have personally replied to all my e-mails and questions. You even gave me ideas regarding removing my old chair. I had a great experience with my transaction; no wonder you have a AAA rating from BBB.org. Your company will be my first choice for my next massage chair.

Thank you.

Mina Chang
Washington

"I knew that I found the right place to purchase our new massage chair."

I was ready to order a massage chair from another online vendor, but after reading your articles, I decided to check them out further through the Better Business Bureau. Needless to say, they had a few blemishes on their record, which was enough for me not to purchase through them. My budget for a new massage chair was $1,600 to $2,000 initially. But after much research online (where it was difficult to find unbiased opinions), I increased to $3,000.

Thanks to your wonderful staff, I was greeted so cheerfully by Stephanie, who answered all of my questions and promptly checked on price matching and shipping time. I knew that I found the right place to purchase our new massage chair. I just thought you should know how much I appreciate the time and effort you have put into your research and for sharing it with consumers like me who do not have access otherwise to trying out the chairs before we purchase. Thank you again for all of your help. We cannot wait to receive our new Panasonic massage chair.

Sincerely,
Lynn Dettman
Green Bay, WI

"I checked out many places before I ordered, and you were both the least expensive and had the most information!"

Thank you so very much for making my purchase of the Human Touch Massage Chair so easy! From the beginning to end, your contact and support were wonderful! The chair arrived perfectly and exactly when they said it would. I have fibromyalgia and massage is one thing that helps ease my pain, but it is time consuming and expensive to go for a massage every day. I put our new chair in the living room, and we have used it every day. My husband and sons all use it too and think it's wonderful. Your website is wonderful, and the free gifts were very useful. Please feel free to use this message on your site as testimony from a satisfied customer! You are the best! I checked out many places before I ordered, and you were both the least expensive and had the most information!

THANK YOU!!
Barb Vittetoe

"I could not be happier with the service and the product!"

Service was great....I was constantly informed of the order progress and where the chair was in the delivery. The chair was delivered to my house, carried up the stairs, then set up ready to use. I could not be happier with the service and the product.

Jerry Horton

Dr. Weidner,

I wanted to take a moment to compliment you on your customer service to date. I have been working as an executive assistant for almost 30 years and in recent years have found that customer service has deteriorated significantly. Your company, on the other hand, is providing first-rate customer service from the initial order process to the delivery updates. I ordered this chair for my boss's son; perhaps one day, I will be in a position to order one for myself (smile).

Thank you for making my job easier. My best to you and your future successes. Regards,

Donna Peart

I am enjoying my massage chair. After a day seeing children as a pediatrician, it's great to come home to a relaxing massage. I have some arthritis in my hip, and the stretching really helps with the pain. Thank you for doing what you said you would do every step of the way, including reasonable pricing, shipping, gifts, availability, response to questions, and warranty paperwork. I can recommend your business with highest regards without reservation. Thank you.

Elliot Feit, MD
Fellow American Academy of Pediatrics
Atlanta, Georgia

Dr. Weidner,

The two chairs I ordered were delivered last Friday, and we have been enjoying them immensely for the past three days. When your website indicated free shipping, I expected the chairs would take two or three weeks to arrive. I never expected them to be air-freighted here in a matter of a couple days.

The Human Touch chairs are fantastic—we're reluctant to show them to our friends as we suspect they won't leave and go home.

Bob Stewart
Boulder, CO

I am VERY impressed with your system and your customer service. As a business owner, I recognize the importance of good after-sale follow-up. I like how you are proactive and let your clients know what to expect well in advance. I also really liked your staff and your online 'chat' capability.

Because of all of this, I will buy things from you again.

Jeff Salisbury
Orange, California

Hello, Dr. Weidner,

I wanted to let you know that...we got the chair really fast and are very happy with it! We thank you for the fantastic service and great help on the phone.

Thank you! Great service!

Astrid Janssen
Stroudsburg, Pennsylvania

Hello, Alan,

As you know, we had quite a time getting delivery of our Interactive Health 1650 as they (not you) delayed our shipping for 17 days. But without your help, we would never have gotten our chair before Christmas. The Interactive Health 1650 is worth the price. It should be reminded to customers that the footrest must be fully reclined to operate, but otherwise you were right that it is very easy to use. Thanks again. We would not shop anywhere else.

Wally Schroeder
Arizona

Dr. Alan Weidner-

Received the HT-140 Massage chair in approximately a week. Love it! Couldn't unpack and set it up fast enough. The delivery person brought the chair to the door, and my three-year-old grandson was quite anxious to help me unpack it. I do massage therapy and somehow missed out on getting a massage myself. I took care of everyone else and forgot about myself. All the features have proven very relaxing to tense muscles and stiffness. My husband and I use it every day. This chair is certainly the best Christmas gift my husband and I decided to get for each other. My son and daughter-in-law were fighting to get on it first. I am sure Christmas Day, the teenage grandchildren, who are very active in sports, will also be fighting for their turn. Never bought anything over the Internet before and were a bit leery with making this purchase. We are so glad we made the decision to go ahead and order it. Appreciated the e-mail updates as the shipment was processed. Thank you so much for the opportunity to enjoy this chair, hopefully for many years and in good health.

Janet Bender

A few months ago, I was looking for the perfect birthday present for my husband. He always complained of backaches and dreamed of a massage chair. I found this website but had many hesitations in placing an order because we live in Germany. After a few very encouraging e-mails between Dr. Alan Weidner and myself, I decided to go through with the order for the HT-125. I received absolutely incredible customer service from the minute I sent the first mail until after the chair was delivered. Dr. Weidner helped me with import customs questions and supplied the transformer that converted the electricity for the chair when it got to Europe. Since this was a surprise present for my husband, it had to be delivered on or shortly before his birthday. I was constantly updated regarding the shipping status to assure an on-time delivery here in Stuttgart.

After the chair arrived (exactly perfect timing, by the way), I was so relieved that it made it all the way here in one piece. My husband was absolutely surprised and very happy to see his gift. He tried it out right away. Unfortunately, he found something wrong with the electronics. A few programs weren't working. I was so disappointed. It was my worst nightmare. What would I do now with a broken massage chair? Send it back to the U.S.? I immediately sent Dr. Alan Weidner an e-mail asking for help, and he responded promptly with a solution. The problem happened most likely during transportation and had to do with the electronics in the back of the chair. Although the parts are not covered under warranty when the chair leaves the U.S., Dr. Weidner shipped us the replacement parts completely free of charge. If that isn't incredible customer service, I don't know what is. The instructions that were sent with the replacement part were easy to follow, and we completed the repair ourselves. My husband and I both use the massage chair and couldn't be happier about the purchase.

Erika Kaercher
Stuttgart, Germany

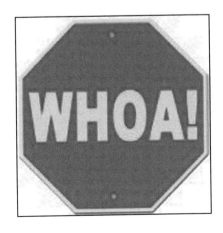

d) Contraindications for Massage Therapy

Although massage therapy is obviously a great therapy for people of all ages, there are also some contraindications of massage. If you have any of the following conditions, please consult with a doctor to confirm that massage will be OK for you.

I might just add that although diabetes is on the list, my type 1 diabetic 27-year-old daughter uses massage chairs regularly without any negative consequences.

Also, when cancer is mentioned, my training as a chiropractor taught us not to apply massage to a part of the body that has a cancerous tumor. However, if you have cancer in a body location distant from the areas that the chair will apply massage therapy, you are probably OK to use the chair. I have a recent customer who has liver cancer, and his oncologist said it was fine to use a massage chair. So, again, consult with your doc if you have any of these conditions or if you have any other concerns about using a massage chair with your medical condition.

Contraindications can be local or complete. *Local* means that in certain situations, massage may still be indicated depending on the locale of the condition. *Complete* generally means that it is definitely a no-no to apply massage therapy. Again, if you are not sure or are concerned about using a massage chair in any of these situations, consult with your doc. Here is the list (taken from http://massage.ca/contraindictionscautions.html):

Local Contraindications:

Acute inflammation

Broken bone/over a nonconsolidating fracture

Recent surgery

Inflammation of the skin

Varicosities (varicose veins) over sites with deep vein thrombosis

Local contagious conditions

Blood clots

Open wound or sore

Local irritable skin conditions

Undiagnosed lump

Acute lesion

Malignancy/active cancer

Skin infection

Tumor

Acute flare-up of rheumatoid arthritis

Recent burn

Phlebitis (inflammation of a vein)

Phlebothrombosis (blood clots in the veins)

Arteritis (inflammation of the arteries)

Complete Contraindications:

Burns (severe)
Infectious disease
Anaphylaxis (life-threatening allergic reaction)
Appendicitis (painful inflamed appendix)
Cerebrocardiovascular accident (stroke)
Insulin shock or diabetic coma
Epileptic seizure (convulsions)
Myocardial infarction (heart attack)
Pneumothorax (air or gas within the chest cavity around the lung)
Atelectasis (a collapsed portion of the lung that does not contain air)
Severe asthmatic attack

Syncope (fainting or loss of consciousness)

Acute pneumonia

Advanced kidney failure, respiratory failure, or liver failure (a very modified treatment may be possible with medical consent)

Diabetic complications such as gangrene, advanced heart or kidney disease, or very unstable high blood pressure

Eclampsia (a severe form {life-threatening} of pregnancy-induced hypertension resulting in seizures)

Hemophilia severe type (a hereditary bleeding disorder)

Hemorrhage (involves rapid and uncontrollable loss of blood)

Arthrosclerosis (severe forms of stiffening or hardening of the joints

Hypertension (unstable) (conditions that are not stable, i.e., post-stroke or heart attack)

Medical shock (a life-threatening medical emergency and one of the leading causes of death for critically ill people; the body reacts and produces insufficient blood flow to reach the body tissues)

Fever above 38.5 degree C or 101.5 F (significant)

Some highly metastatic cancers (diagnosed not to be terminal)

Systemic contagious or infectious conditions

This list is from a website for massage therapists. Of course, a massage chair is different from the actual hands of a massage therapist, so some of these conditions may not necessarily be subject to the same caution as would be a massage therapist. Again, if concerned or in doubt, consult with your physician.

e) Massage Chair Resources

Here is my list of resources that I use and should assist you in massage chair research, shipping, and repairs:

1. **Comparison Chart** – It took me three to four months to put this resource together for my customers, and, to this day, it is the most viewed page on my website next to the home page. You can compare over 50 features of any of the models we carry. It is a great tool for

your research and will give you a good feeling for what each chair has available.

http://www.massage-chair-relief.com/massage-chair-comparison/

As good as a tool that the chart is, there is nothing like sitting in a chair to experience it and knowing for sure if it is right for you. You can always do that by visiting our showroom…

2. **Massage Chair Relief Showroom** – At the time of this writing, our showroom is the only one of its kind in the country where a shopper can try out all the major name brands under one roof. I know Salt Lake City is not a convenient place for the rest of the country, but we have a program in place to help you get here. It's called the Out-of-Stater program and will make it possible for you to come visit us for next to nothing. The following link explains how it works:

http://www.massage-chair-relief.com/out-of-state.html

3. **YouTube Channel** – We have a YouTube channel with hundreds of videos, all designed to assist you, the massage chair shopper, with making the all-important decision about which chair is right for you. I put up one to three videos every week on all topics related to massage chairs. At the present time, we have the following categories on the channel:

a) *Massage Chair Industry Updates* – Every two weeks, I put out a 10–15 minute video in which I discuss the latest news and notes in the massage chair industry. You can be updated about new models, discontinued models, stock status, sales, and much more.

b) *Massage Chair Feature Reviews* – We take a chair model and break down each feature into a short two- to five-minute video that demonstrates how that feature works. This is very helpful for people who cannot get to the showroom and need more of a hands-on display of a chair and its features.

c) *Massage Chair Industry Interviews* – From time to time, I interview heads of massage chair companies and other industry experts to get the latest insights from those in the know. Many times, we learn about the inner workings of a massage chair company through these interviews. Some of the videos involve a visit by me to their headquarters, their inventory warehouse, or their showrooms to really see what is going on in these companies.

d) *Massage Chair Dictionary* – We take the terms from our chapter on the massage chair glossary and put them to video so that we can visually demonstrate what the term means.

e) *Massage-Chair-Relief.com Tutorials* – These are on-screen video tutorials that walk the user through various tasks on our website, making it easier to navigate our very large site.

Naturally, I strongly recommend that you subscribe to our **YouTube channel** so that you can be notified the moment we put up a new video. You can go to our channel through this link:

http://www.youtube.com/massagechairrelief

4. **Article Library/Blog** – We have the largest collection of articles in the massage chair industry. You can find pretty much anything you want as it pertains to this industry through our very extensive article library. Here is a link to that collection:

http://www.massage-chair-relief.com/blog/

You can search for any topic in the search bar located on the right-hand side of any page of our article library.

5. **Massage Chair Reviews** – Massage Chair Relief has the largest collection of massage chair reviews in the business…and these are real reviews from real people! Go to any product page on the site and you will see a section called "Reviews." These reviews will help

you immensely in getting honest feedback about a model you may be interested in.

6. **Shipping Companies** – As you can imagine, we do a lot of shipping in our business and have used many different shipping companies along the way. Most people think of UPS when they want to ship something. Well, UPS does have a freight department, but they can be a bit expensive (and massage chairs are already expensive to ship because of their weight and size).

Here is a list of companies we have used in the past who may be able to give you some pricing options should you want to sell your chair or if you have purchased one from outside of your state that will require some long-haul shipping:

a) YRC – http://www.yrc.com

b) Roadrunner – http://www.rrts.com

c) Diamond – http://www.diamondshipping.com

d) TechTrans – http://www.techtrans.com

e) UPS Freight – http://www.upsfreight.com

f) Nonstop Delivery – http://www.nonstopdelivery.com

All of the above-mentioned companies have shipped for us in the past. If you want to also arrange white glove delivery for your chair, Tech Trans and Nonstop Delivery offer that option.

6. **Massage Chair Repairs** – A lot of folks like to do their own repairs. The massage chair companies will help you diagnose any problem over the phone and send you the part(s) you need. But what if you are like me and have no "handyman genes" in your body? What do you do when your chair is out of warranty?

Most massage chair companies outsource the labor portion of their warranty to a third-party company. The company most commonly used is Jez Enterprises (there are others). They have a national network of technicians who are deployed by the massage chair companies as needed to repair your massage chair.

If your chair is out of warranty, you can still give Jez Enterprises a call to find someone in your area who can come and work on your chair. Of course, you can still get all your parts from the massage chair company itself, but Jez Enterprises is a good choice for a local tech to come out to your home or business to do the labor.

Here is Jez Enterprises' contact info...

http://www.jezinc.com

2308 E Kiehl Ave, Sherwood, AR 72120

(501) 835-2095

7. Massage Chair Company Contact Information

    a) Inada
        http://wwwinadausa.com
        888-769-0555
        2125 32nd Street, Boulder, CO 80301

    b) Human Touch
        http://www.humantouch.com

        866-369-9426
        3030 Walnut Avenue, Long Beach, CA 90807

    c) Infinite Therapeutics
        http://www.infinitetherapeutics.com

603-347-6006
68A Route 125 • Kingston, NH 03848

d) Osaki
http://www.osakimassagechair.com
888-848-2630
1721 N. Central Expy., Plano, TX 75075

e) Luraco
http://www.luraco.com
800-483-9930
1132 107th Street, Arlington, TX 76011

f) Omega
http://www.omegamassage.com
800-659-3650
4065 East La Palma Avenue, Suite D, Anaheim, CA 92807

g) Cozzia
http://www.cozziausa.com
877-977-0656
14331 E Don Julian Rd, City of Industry, CA 91746

h) Panasonic
http://www.panasonic.com

About the Author

Dr. Alan Weidner is a 1991 summa cum laude graduate of the Los Angeles College of Chiropractic. Originally from Edmonton, Alberta, Canada, Dr. Weidner immigrated to the USA in 1988 to attend school and pursue his career.

He settled in Utah upon graduating and practiced in his own clinic for seventeen years before selling the practice and opening the Massage Chair Relief brick-and-mortar showroom in 2009. His showroom is the only one of its kind in the country. There, you can find all the major name-brand chairs under one roof. He has customers who travel from all over the country to test out the massage chairs in his showroom before making a buying decision.

Dr. Weidner actually began selling massage chairs online in July 2005, when he launched www.massage-chair-relief.com. He had an older but well-made Human Touch chair in the clinic for a couple of years before beginning the website. His patients loved the chair and commented to him how it had helped them with their pain symptoms.

Through his clinic newsletter, Dr. Weidner mentioned that if anyone was interested in getting a chair for their home just like the one he had in his clinic, he could get it for a very good price. He had two buyers. Both were patients who used to come quite regularly, every few weeks, to the clinic for pain relief. He noticed, however, that after selling them the chairs, he did not see them for quite some time. After about six months, he spoke with his neighbor whose daughter had purchased one of the chairs and asked him why she didn't come back to the clinic for treatments anymore. The neighbor told Dr. Weidner that it was because his daughter's chair took care of most of her discomfort. When the second buyer finally came back to the clinic, she said the same thing…that the chair had taken care of most of her pain.

Dr. Weidner started looking into making the sale of massage chairs an adjunct business to his chiropractic office. That is how the massage chair business essentially started. Dr. Weidner checked into the viability of marketing massage chairs in his clinic, but it seemed like it was almost impossible to find good information on the differences among the various massage chairs out there…and that there were far too many cheapo massage chair companies flooding the market with low-quality (and sometimes even dangerous) knockoffs… knockoffs that Dr. Weidner wouldn't feel comfortable using himself or recommending to his patients.

As a chiropractic doctor with a deep understanding of the human body and how it interacts with these chairs, Dr. Weidner wanted to make his way through the confusing double-talk and marketing hype and make a decision about what chairs would be best for his clinic (and what chairs he would feel comfortable recommending to his patients). His clinic became a showroom of sorts for the models he had on display for his patients, but the vast majority of his sales were through his website, which quickly became one of the top online massage chair websites in the industry.

After his first full year of selling massage chairs online (2006), Dr. Weidner put his practice up for sale so that he could devote 100% of his time to the massage chair business. It became his passion. It took two years for the practice to finally sell, but in June 2008, he opened his Massage Chair Relief showroom in the very same strip mall where he had practiced for seventeen years…just five doors down!

Today, Dr. Weidner is the most recognized face in the massage chair industry and continues to be a prolific educator and champion for the massage chair consumer. His articles and video tutorials have been the primary source of education for thousands of shoppers.

Dr. Weidner is married and the father of six wonderful children and a growing brood of grandchildren. He still plays ice hockey regularly, which has made him a very faithful massage chair user!

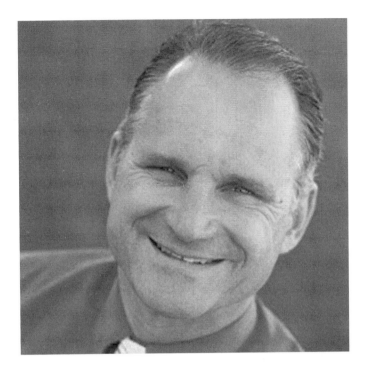

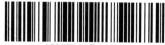
Made in the USA
San Bernardino, CA
13 October 2014